THE
ELDERLY CRISIS

WHO WILL BE THERE WHEN THEY NEED US THE MOST

Preparing for an Aging Population: A wake-up call for more solutions to a society that has been overlooked

NORMA CARBY

Copyright

The Elderly Crisis: Who Will Be There When They Need Us The Most

Copyright © 2025 Norma Carby

City of Publication: New Rochelle, NY

Made and Printed in the United States of America

All rights reserved. No part of this book may be reproduced, distributed, or transmitted in any form or by any means, including photocopying, recording, or other electronic or mechanical methods, without the prior written permission of the publisher or copyright holder, except in the case of brief quotations embodied in critical reviews and certain other noncommercial uses permitted by copyright law.

Library of Congress Control Number: 2025909826

ISBN: 979-8-9989059-0-2 Paperback

ISBN: 979-8-9989059-1-9 Hardcover

First Edition: 2025

Moral Rights of the Author

The author of this work has asserted their moral rights to be identified as the author of this work in accordance with the Copyright, Designs and Patents Act (United Kingdom). The author also asserts their right to be recognized as the author of this publication under the applicable laws of the United States of America.

Disclaimer:

This book provides information and insights on the topic of the elderly crisis. It is not intended to provide medical, legal, financial, or other professional advice. Readers should consult with qualified professionals for specific guidance related to their individual circumstances. The author and publisher disclaim any liability for any actions taken based on the information provided in this book.

Normaknowz LLC

New Rochelle, NY

www.normaknowz.com

DEDICATION

This book is dedicated to my mother, Cecelia Veronica Carby, who passed away in November 2024 after a courageous battle with Alzheimer's. A devoted mother of three, the heart of the family, her sacrifices paved the way for a better life for her children. Mum's strength, resilience, and unwavering belief in doing one's best will forever be my guiding light. She faced life's challenges with extraordinary grace, teaching me invaluable lessons. This book is a testament to her influence to persevere, to strive for my best, and to always trust in God. Her legacy lives on through these pages.

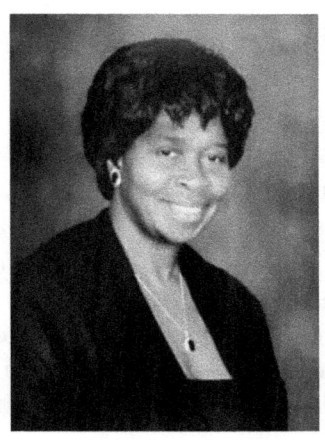

ACKNOWLEDGEMENTS

To my dearest brother, Stephen Carby, words cannot express the depth of my gratitude. Sharing the care of Mum with you was a true gift. Your unwavering support, not just as a brother, but as a father figure and role model, meant the world to me. I'm filled with pride for the way we came together, providing Mum with the most loving care imaginable. We did it, Stephen. And as I write this, tears of love and appreciation fill my eyes, knowing we couldn't have done it without each other. Thank you for showing the world, and me, the true meaning of brotherhood.

To Michael Carby, my younger brother: this first Mother's Day without Mum finds me especially mindful of the solace and strength we draw from one another. Your presence, today and always, is a cherished reminder of the enduring power of family. Your accomplishments are a source of immense pride, a reflection of the values we were raised with, and a tribute to Mum's legacy.

I want to acknowledge my dear friend, Julie Johns, a fellow full-time caregiver for her mum. For 35 years, we've shared life's joys and challenges, never imagining we'd find ourselves on this parallel path of elder care. Hailing from the UK, just like me, Julie has been an incredible source of support, understanding the emotional and physical rollercoaster of this journey. We've laughed, we've cried, we've leaned on each other through thick and thin. Thank you, Julie, for your unwavering friendship and for your invaluable contributions to this book.

It is with profound gratitude that I also wish to acknowledge

Evangeline Myrie, affectionately known to our family as "Sister Myrie," a cherished, longtime friend and devoted fellow church sister of my dear mum. Evangeline played an absolutely indispensable role during my mum's final months, proving to be a true beacon of strength and unwavering support that extended far beyond mere phone calls.

Evangeline graced our home on several occasions, bringing solace and spiritual comfort through her fervent prayers and the beautiful hymns she sang to my mum. Those prayers, so deeply felt, and those songs, so divinely inspired, were a profound source of peace and exactly what my mum, a true servant of God who lived to attend church and worship Him, so greatly needed.

And for me, in those trying times, your selfless acts of bringing nourishing food ensured I was eating and caring for myself. This was a testament to your boundless compassion, a truly selfless devotion you extended to both of us. Right up until my mum's very last days, your steadfast presence was a comforting anchor. The entire Carby family will be eternally grateful for your invaluable time, your generous giving, and your unwavering commitment to us during such a tender period. Thank you, from the depths of our hearts.

For the presentation and structure of this book, I extend my deepest gratitude to my exceptionally gifted and talented friend, Constance Banks. Her unwavering commitment to this project proved absolutely instrumental in bringing it to fruition. I am profoundly grateful for her truly invaluable assistance; she was, without a doubt, the destiny helper God divinely provided along my path. It has been an absolute pleasure to work with Constance, and her meticulous attention to detail has been nothing short of transformative, playing an indispensable role in shaping this book into the impactful work it is today. Her insightful contributions have enriched its very essence, and I am grateful to her for her dedication and expertise. Therefore, I offer my sincere gratitude and thanks to Constance.

LETTER TO GOD

Father, thank you for teaching me and showing me the way of your word. It states in Exodus 20:12, as part of the commandments, "Honor your father and your mother, so that you may live long in the land the Lord your God is giving you." Knowing this, Lord, you have allowed me to take on the responsibility of caring for my mum and honoring her for all she has done for me.

I thank you for giving me the strength and the grace never to give up, and even in the times that things got overwhelming, you strengthened me to press on. It is because of you that my love has been unconditional; it is because of you that I have excelled in compassion, love, gratitude, and the greatest need to pray. Father, through you, all things are possible, and you made it possible for me to take care of my mum. Your word never returns void, and so, my honoring of my mother allowed her to speak blessings over me and for me to know true love. Father, thank you for changing the course of my life to do what is right and also to serve you. I thank you for my mum's life and the time you allowed me to spend with her. I will continue to stay obedient to your word.

Thank you for your amazing love and compassion; you have blessed me, and I remain in the blessing for your namesake; Amen.

TABLE OF CONTENTS

Chapter 1: A Crisis Ignored: Unveiling the True Scope of Elder Neglect..................13

Chapter 2: The Breaking Point: When Caregiving Crushes Both Spirit and Body..................31

Chapter 3: Home Truths: The Difficulties Elders Face Within Families..................47

Chapter 4: Systems That Fail: When Nations and the World Abandon Their Elders..................57

Chapter 5: The Price of Dignity: How Finances Shatter the Dream of a Secure Old Age..................65

Chapter 6: A Call to Action: Reclaiming Humanity for Our Forgotten Generation..................71

Chapter 7: Coming Together: Creating a Supportive World for Seniors..................85

Chapter 8: Our Legacy of Love: Building a World Where No Elder Stands Alone..................93

Closing Summary..................100

DESCRIPTION

As our loved ones grow older, the question of their care becomes increasingly urgent. "The Elderly Crisis" delves into the heart of this issue, exploring the emotional, financial, and societal challenges facing seniors and their families. Through compelling stories and insightful analysis, this book shines a light on the often-overlooked needs of our aging population and calls for a compassionate and comprehensive approach to elder care.

INTRODUCTION

This book was born from a desire to share my intimate journey of caring for my mother full-time. It's a story of learning to truly understand her needs, along with navigating the complexities of doctors, healthcare facilities, and agencies, and ultimately, discovering the profound rewards and unexpected challenges of such a commitment. If you've ever wondered what it's like to care for a loved one through their aging years, if you're seeking to understand the emotional rollercoaster and practical considerations for both parent and caregiver, then please, settle in with a cup of tea, and let's begin.

A few years ago, I made a life-altering decision to move back home and care for Mum. At the time, I didn't fully grasp that it would mean surrendering my own plans, my lifestyle, essentially, my entire sense of normalcy. Some days were pleasantly pleasing, and gentle, filled with great pleasure, but many were incredibly demanding. Eight hours of uninterrupted sleep became a distant memory, as my world revolved around Mum's well-being and meeting her needs. She had been diagnosed with early-onset Alzheimer's shortly after completing her double Master's degree, a cruel twist of fate that began around the age of 68.

Caring for a loved one is an act of profound commitment, often requiring a level of selflessness that can feel overwhelming. Yet, I found solace in remembering the countless ways Mum cared for me when I was a child, utterly dependent on her. The tables had simply turned, as they inevitably do.

Having spent my childhood in England, immersed in a predominantly white community, I was accustomed to seeing grandmothers living contentedly within the family home. When we moved to America, I encountered a culture that often prioritized the hustle of individual pursuits, with less emphasis on extended family care. Looking back, I'm deeply grateful for those early years in England, as they instilled in me the values that would eventually guide my care for Mum.

"Why me?" was a question that sometimes echoed in my mind. But then, I'd remember the West Indian culture that shaped my upbringing, where caring for our elders within the family was an unspoken commandment. Mum had taught me well, embedding within me the principles that solidified my decision to care for her myself, along with my brother Steve. In doing so, I discovered a deeper sense of purpose, a significance I hadn't known before. Mum gave me countless gifts, but perhaps the greatest was the opportunity to love more deeply, to embrace selflessness, and to place my complete trust in God. The need to be seen or heard faded in the light of this profound responsibility.

My hope is that within these pages, you will find resonance with your own experiences, perhaps discovering a renewed sense of purpose. If you're facing the daunting decision of whether or not to care for a loved one yourself, I hope this book offers you clarity, guidance, and the courage to follow your heart.

The Elderly Crisis

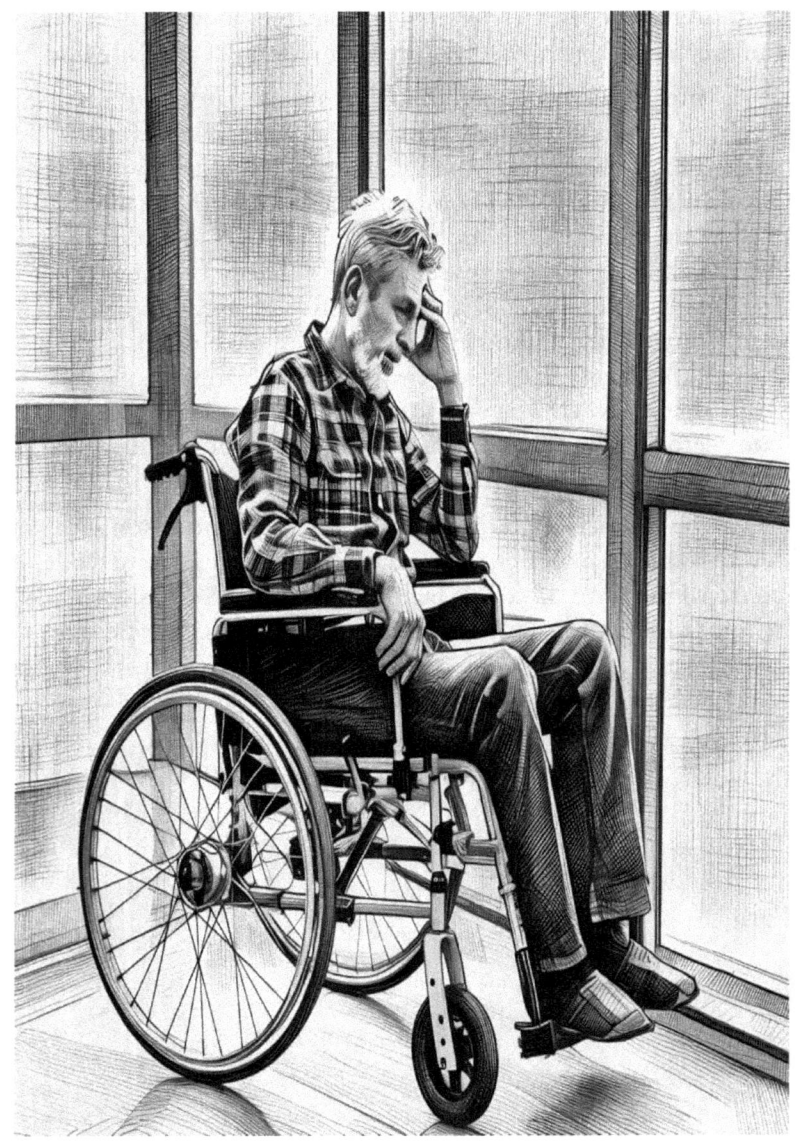

Chapter 1

A Crisis Ignored: Unveiling the True Scope of Elder Neglect

The elderly face a multitude of significant issues today.
Loneliness and Isolation:
As people age, the loss of friends and family can trigger deep feelings of loneliness and isolation. Depression, often a silent consequence of this isolation, can further prevent seniors from communicating their needs and seeking help. Reduced mobility and decreased social engagement can exacerbate these feelings, creating a challenging cycle. The body naturally slows down, impacting independence and making it difficult to ask for help, sometimes leading to seniors feeling like a burden. Caregivers, too, can experience loneliness and isolation, as their full attention is often consumed by caring for their loved one. My own time became increasingly limited as Mum's Alzheimer's progressed, requiring constant companionship. While it's often said that caregivers need breaks, and this is absolutely true, every moment I spent with Mum felt like a blessing, regardless of the challenges. My brother's daily support was invaluable, allowing us to depend on each other when needed. This highlights the importance of family support and open communication. Never assume everything is fine just because it's not discussed. Companionship is essential for seniors. Family meetings can provide a platform to discuss these often-unspoken issues and create a plan to combat loneliness.

Here are some ideas to consider:

Regular visits: Schedule consistent visits from family

members, friends, or volunteers.

- **Social Activities:** Encourage participation in senior centers, community groups, or religious organizations.
- **Technology Connection:** Help seniors utilize video calls, social media, or email to stay connected with loved ones.
- **Pet Companionship:** If appropriate, consider adopting a pet to provide companionship and emotional support.
- **Respite Care:** Utilize respite care services to give caregivers a break and provide seniors with social interaction.
- **Meaningful Activities:** Engage seniors in hobbies, crafts, or other activities that bring them joy and a sense of purpose.

Nursing homes should be a last resort. Strive to create a supportive environment at home, ensuring your loved one feels valued and connected, and not like just a number.

Ageism:

Aging is a natural part of life, a journey we all share. Yet, in a society that often prioritizes youth, the realities of growing older can be met with anxiety and even fear, regardless of age. While aging brings wisdom and a wealth of lived experience, it also presents unique challenges. Physical changes, such as declining mobility and health issues, can impact independence and well-being. Cognitive changes, including memory loss, can be particularly distressing. And the emotional landscape of aging, marked by potential losses and transitions, can lead to feelings of isolation and vulnerability. Witnessing my mum's journey with aging brought this reality home for me, not just as her caregiver, but as someone navigating my own aging process. It's a deeply personal experience, one that shifts our perspective on what it means to "look young" and "feel young." We observe aging in others but recognizing it within ourselves requires a different kind of awareness, a gentle slowing down that allows life to unfold at its own pace.

It's crucial to acknowledge that aging is not a monolithic experience. Every individual ages differently, with varying needs and strengths. However, some common concerns facing the elderly include:

- **Physical Health:** Managing chronic conditions, navigating healthcare systems, and maintaining physical function become increasingly important.

- **Mental and Emotional Health:** Addressing depression, anxiety, loneliness, and age-related cognitive changes is vital for overall well-being.

- **Social Connection:** Combating isolation through social engagement, meaningful activities, and intergenerational connections is essential.

- **Financial Security:** Ensuring access to resources, managing retirement income, and planning for long-term care needs are critical.

- **Autonomy and Independence:** Supporting seniors' ability to make choices, maintain control over their lives, and age with dignity is paramount.

Unfortunately, ageism, or discrimination based on age, remains a pervasive issue. It can manifest in subtle ways, from patronizing language to limited access to services and opportunities. Ageism not only devalues the elderly but also perpetuates harmful stereotypes that can negatively impact their self-esteem and well-being. Let us remember that we are all aging, every single day. By choosing kindness and inclusivity, we can ensure that no one, at any age, feels overlooked or undervalued.

There are numerous resources available to support seniors and their families worldwide:

- **Government Programs are Available in Most Countries:** For the US, Medicare, Social Security, and other federal and state programs offer vital assistance with healthcare, income, and support services (limited but available).
- **Non-profit Organizations:** The National Council on Aging, the AARP, and other organizations provide resources, advocacy, and support for seniors.
- **Local Agencies on Aging:** These community-based organizations offer a range of services, including transportation, meals, home care, and senior centers.
- **Area Agencies on Aging (AAAs):** These agencies provide information and assistance with accessing resources for seniors and people with disabilities.
- **Senior Centers:** These community hubs offer social activities, educational programs, and opportunities for engagement.
- **Online Resources:** Websites like the National Institute on Aging (NIA) and the Eldercare Locator provide valuable information and tools.

As a society, we all have a role to play in supporting our aging population. It starts with simple yet profound actions. Putting away our phones and prioritizing quality time with loved ones can make a significant difference. Exploring local church programs that serve seniors is another wonderful way to get involved. Even something as basic as neighbor awareness; knowing who lives on your street and checking in on them can have a huge impact. These small gestures of connection can combat isolation and foster a sense of community.

But we must also address the broader issues facing our aging population. We need to challenge ageism, speaking out against ageist attitudes and stereotypes and promoting positive, realistic images of aging. Creating truly age-friendly communities where seniors feel valued and respected is essential. This includes supporting intergenerational programs that bridge the gap between generations.

On a practical level, we can offer assistance with transportation, errands, home maintenance, or other daily tasks that may become challenging. Staying connected through regular visits, calls, and engaging conversations is vital for combating social isolation, a silent epidemic among the elderly.

We must also advocate for change, supporting policies and programs that benefit seniors and raising awareness about the challenges of aging. And perhaps most importantly, we must listen and learn from the wisdom and experience of older adults, creating opportunities for them to share their stories and knowledge.

By recognizing the diverse needs of our aging population, challenging ageism, and actively supporting seniors and their families, we can create a society where everyone ages with dignity, respect, and connection. I've witnessed the power of this firsthand in my own neighborhood. Living on a quiet street with several residents over 100 years old, I've seen how small acts of caring and neighborly support can make a world of difference. It truly does take a village, and it's a responsibility we all share, because, as we know, we are all going to get old.

Healthcare Costs:

Healthcare costs in retirement can be a major concern, often stretching already tight budgets. While long-term care and prescription drugs rightly command attention, it's the everyday expenses that often catch seniors off guard. Think about it: doctor's visits, specialist co-pays, hospital stays, even with insurance, can add up quickly. Dental and vision care, often not fully covered by Medicare or similar international programs, can create significant out-of-pocket burdens. Hearing aids, crucial for staying connected, can be surprisingly expensive. And what about the ongoing costs of medical equipment, like walkers or diabetic supplies? Plus, transportation to appointments and over-the-counter medications are recurring expenses that can strain a fixed income.

Here's the good news:

While these costs can feel overwhelming, there are proactive steps you can take. Consider supplementing your existing coverage with individual policies designed for healthcare needs in retirement. If you're still working, explore options for additional coverage through your employer's plan.

But perhaps the most important step of all is to have a **dedicated advocate**, whether it's a family member or trusted individual, who can stay on top of your healthcare needs.

Aging often comes with forgetfulness, making it easy to lose track of appointments, follow-up care, test results, and referrals. The healthcare system, unfortunately, doesn't always take the initiative to ensure seamless care for seniors. It takes a proactive advocate to fill that gap.

Choose a family advocate who can attend doctor's visits with you, take detailed notes, and ask questions. This advocate can help ensure that test results are received promptly, appointments are scheduled and kept, and referrals to specialists are followed through. They can also research treatment options, compare costs, and advocate for your best interests when dealing with insurance companies and healthcare providers.

From personal experience, I can't stress enough how vital this role is.

Whether it was a doctor's appointment, a medical test, or coordinating additional services, I had to be constantly involved, often "walking behind" the doctors and nurses to ensure things were done correctly and efficiently. I also made sure to educate myself thoroughly on my loved one's conditions and treatment options, so I could be an informed and effective advocate.

Planning ahead, including securing additional coverage and choosing a dedicated healthcare advocate, can make a world of difference in protecting your health and financial well-being in your golden years.

Financial Insecurity:

Financial Insecurity is a harsh reality for many seniors. Inadequate retirement savings, rising living costs, and unexpected medical expenses can create a perfect storm, leaving individuals struggling to maintain a decent standard of living. This financial strain can lead to significant stress, anxiety, and a diminished quality of life.

One common misconception is that seniors who come from backgrounds of limited resources are destined to be financially insecure. In fact, some seniors who have experienced financial hardship earlier in life develop a strong sense of thrift and a desire to provide for their children. However, this admirable intention can sometimes lead them to prioritize leaving an inheritance over adequately preparing for their own long-term needs. It's crucial to strike a balance between supporting loved ones and ensuring one's own financial security in later years.

Another harmful stereotype is the assumption that elderly individuals are inherently unable to manage their finances. While cognitive decline can affect financial decision-making for some, many seniors are perfectly capable of handling their own affairs. The key is to empower them with the knowledge and resources they need to make informed choices.

Taking control of your finances is an act of self-care that directly contributes to your well-being later in life.

It's about investing in yourself, ensuring that your needs are met, and reducing the potential burden on your family or social support systems.

My mother, having witnessed the vulnerabilities of relying solely on external systems during her time as a nurse, understood the importance of financial independence in aging. She prioritized saving and planning, ensuring she had options and control over her care in her senior years. This proactive approach allowed her to navigate her later years with greater peace of mind.

Preparing financially for the future requires a shift in mindset.

It's about recognizing that relying solely on government programs or family support may not be enough. It's about taking ownership of your financial well-being and making conscious choices that will benefit you in the long run.

Here are some concrete steps you can take to prepare financially for what may lie ahead:

- **Create a Realistic Budget:** Track your income and expenses to identify areas where you can save. Even small adjustments can make a big difference over time.

- **Maximize Retirement Savings:** Contribute the maximum amount to your 401(k), IRA, or other retirement accounts. If your employer offers a matching contribution, take advantage of it.

- **Seek Professional Financial Advice:** A financial advisor can help you develop a personalized retirement plan, taking into account your specific circumstances and goals.

- **Explore Long-Term Care Insurance:** Long-term care insurance can help cover the high costs of assisted living, nursing home care, or in-home care. It's generally more affordable to purchase this type of insurance in your 50s or 60s.

- **Invest Wisely:** Consider diversifying your

investments to balance risk and potential returns. Educate yourself about different investment options or work with a financial advisor.

- **Manage Debt:** Pay down high-interest debt, such as credit card debt, as quickly as possible. Reducing your debt burden can free up more money for saving and investing.

- **Plan for Healthcare Costs:** Research Medicare options and consider supplemental insurance to help cover out-of-pocket expenses. Factor in the potential costs of prescription drugs, dental care, vision care, and hearing aids.

- **Create an Emergency Fund:** Set aside a readily accessible fund to cover unexpected expenses, such as medical bills or home repairs.

- **Review and Update Your Plan Regularly:** Your financial plan should be a living document that you review and update periodically to reflect changes in your circumstances and goals.

By taking these steps, you can empower yourself to age with greater financial security and peace of mind, ensuring that your later years are a time of comfort and independence, not financial strain. Remember, investing in yourself is the best investment you can make.

Technological Challenges:

The rapid evolution of technology presents a unique challenge for many older adults. Navigating a landscape of constant updates, new devices, and unfamiliar interfaces can be daunting, leading to feelings of frustration and inadequacy. This difficulty in using technology can have significant consequences, contributing to social isolation, limiting access to vital information and services, and increasing vulnerability to scams and misinformation.

In many ways, the digital revolution has left seniors behind. While younger generations have grown up immersed in technology, many older adults haven't had the same opportunities for learning and gradual adaptation. They're often expected to simply "go with the flow," despite lacking the foundational knowledge and support. This is further compounded by the fact that many seniors are comfortable with traditional methods of communication and information gathering, like landline phones and printed materials. As one gets older, the desire to learn new things can lessen, not because of diminished capacity, but due to a natural inclination towards familiar routines and a sense of "if it ain't broke, don't fix it."

But technology has immense potential to enhance the lives of older adults. It's about finding the right approach, designing technology with seniors in mind, and providing effective training and support. We need to shift our thinking from expecting seniors to adapt to existing technology to creating technology that adapts to their needs and abilities.

My mum, for example, was quite computer savvy but struggled with the complexities of mobile phones. This wasn't due to a lack of intelligence but rather a difference in design philosophy and user experience. Every time she needed to do more than make a call or turn the phone off, she needed assistance. This highlights the need for a "middle ground" technology designed specifically for seniors, with simplified interfaces and intuitive functionality.

Here are some creative ideas on how technology can help the elderly and how we can effectively teach them:

1. Senior-Friendly Devices and Interfaces:

- **Simplified Smartphones:** Develop smartphones with larger screens, bigger buttons, simplified menus, voice command features, and pre-installed apps for essential tasks like calling, texting, video chatting, and accessing photos.

- **Universal Remotes:** Design universal remotes for televisions and other devices with oversized buttons, minimal functions, and voice control.
- **Smart Home Assistants – Bring it back to basics:** Utilize voice-activated assistants like Alexa or Google Home to control lights, thermostats, appliances, and entertainment systems, making daily tasks easier and safer.

2. **Tailored Training and Support:**
   - **Intergenerational Tech Tutors:** Pair high school or college students with seniors for one-on-one technology tutoring. This benefits both generations, fostering connection and digital literacy. This could also be integrated under an internship program or after school program.
   - **Senior Tech Centers:** Create dedicated spaces in communities where seniors can access computers, receive training, and participate in workshops on topics like online safety, social media, and video calling.
   - **"Tech Toolkits" for Seniors:** Develop easy-to-understand guides and tutorials with large print, clear instructions, and visual aids. Offer these toolkits in print and online formats.
   - **In-Home Tech Support:** Provide in-home assistance for seniors who need help setting up devices, learning new software, or troubleshooting technical issues.

3. **Bridging the Digital Divide:**
   - **Community Technology Classes:** Offer free or low-cost technology classes at libraries, community centers, and senior centers. Focus on practical skills and real-life applications.

- **Online Resources and Tutorials:** Create websites and video tutorials specifically designed for seniors, with clear and concise instructions.
- **Senior-Focused App Development:** Encourage the development of apps tailored to seniors' needs and interests, such as medication reminders, health trackers, brain games, and social networking platforms.

4. **Fostering a Culture of Digital Inclusion:**
   - **Promote the Benefits of Technology:** Highlight the ways technology can enhance seniors' lives, such as staying connected with loved ones, accessing healthcare information, and pursuing hobbies.
   - **Address Fears and Concerns:** Acknowledge seniors' anxieties about technology and provide patient, understanding support. Emphasize online safety and security measures.
   - **Celebrate Successes:** Recognize and celebrate seniors' achievements in learning and using technology, building their confidence and motivation.

By embracing these ideas and working collaboratively, we can empower seniors to fully participate in the digital age, enriching their lives and fostering a more inclusive and connected society.

Caregiver Burden:

The weight of caregiving often falls heavily on the shoulders of family members, creating a significant emotional and financial burden. This burden can be particularly acute when support isn't shared equitably among family members. Too often, one individual, like myself, becomes the primary caregiver, while others lead their lives seemingly untouched by the daily demands of elder care. This imbalance can breed resentment and create rifts within families, just when unity and support are needed the most. Thank God for my older brother Stephen who came by daily and also contributed greatly to mum's care, especially on the weekends.

There's no financial compensation for the hours, days, and years spent caring for a loved one. It's an act of love, pure and simple, a labor often undertaken with the understanding that the rewards lie not in monetary gain but in the intangible realm of honoring a life and reciprocating the care once received. For me, caring for Mum was a calling, a profound act of love that shaped my life in ways I couldn't have imagined. I trusted that the sacrifices I made were part of a larger purpose, a belief that sustained me through the challenging times.

Being a caregiver requires a fundamental shift in perspective. Your time is no longer your own; your priorities realign to center on the needs of your loved one. It demands patience, compassion, and an unwavering commitment to providing the best possible care. For my brother and me, placing Mum's care in someone else's hands was never an option. We were driven by a deep desire to honor her wishes and provide the personal, familiar touch that we believed prolonged her life and brought her comfort.

One of the most overlooked aspects of caregiving is the need for appreciation and respite. Caregivers often pour their heart and soul into their role, sacrificing their own well-being in the process. A simple "thank you," acknowledgment of their efforts, can go a long way in validating their dedication. Unfortunately, as I experienced firsthand, such gestures are not always forthcoming. Caregivers also need breaks, time to recharge and reconnect with their own lives. While I never had that option, and thankfully never experienced burnout, I recognize the vital importance of respite for those in similar situations.

My experience as Mum's caregiver was, without a doubt, the most challenging and rewarding "job" I've ever had. It demanded sacrifices, but it also filled my life with a depth of purpose I had never known. I was able to give Mum the same unwavering care she had fought to give me as a child, a full-circle moment that brought profound meaning to my life.

But caregiving shouldn't have to be a journey undertaken alone. Here are some of the things I did with my brother, that I'd now like to share with you:

- **Open Communication:** Discussing caregiving responsibilities openly and honestly, ensuring everyone understands the needs of the individual and the commitment required.

- **Shared Responsibility:** Dividing caregiving duties equitably, taking into account each family member's strengths and availability.

- **Mutual Support:** Offering emotional and practical support to the primary caregiver, recognizing the toll the role can take.

- **Regular Check-ins:** Scheduling regular family meetings to discuss concerns, address challenges, and ensure the caregiving plan is meeting everyone's needs.

- **Respite Planning:** Making a conscious effort to provide respite for the primary caregiver, whether through rotating responsibilities or utilizing respite care services.

- **Financial Contribution:** Contributing financially to the costs associated with caregiving, easing the burden on the primary caregiver.

Beyond the family unit, systemic changes are needed to better support caregivers. These include:

- **Increased Access to Respite Care:** Expanding funding and availability of respite care services, making them more affordable and accessible.

- **Caregiver Tax Credits and Compensation:** Implementing policies that provide financial relief to caregivers, recognizing the valuable service they provide.

- **Public Awareness Campaigns:** Raising awareness about the challenges of caregiving and promoting the importance of caregiver support.

- **Improved Training and Resources:** Providing caregivers with access to training, education, and support groups to help them navigate the complexities of elder care.

By acknowledging the burdens and celebrating the contributions of caregivers, and by implementing supportive policies and practices, we can create a system that truly values and honors both those who give care and those who receive it.

Our commitment to community well-being extends to our elderly neighbors, both of whom are over a century old. While they benefit from dedicated caregivers, my brother and I consistently make ourselves available to provide supplementary assistance and emergency support. This includes practical aid such as shoveling driveways and pathways during inclement weather, and maintaining garden edges in the summer, thereby ensuring the safety of their caregivers and allowing them to focus on their primary responsibilities.

My brother, Steve, has been particularly instrumental, consistently offering external assistance and providing innovative gadgets that enhance our neighbors' comfort and quality of life. This proactive engagement transcends the traditional family unit, underscoring the vital importance of robust community support. Such efforts are crucial not only for the direct benefit and enhanced well-being of our elderly population but also for providing essential reinforcement to their caregivers, who play an indispensable role in their daily lives. By extending a helping hand beyond immediate family, we foster a stronger, more resilient community that collectively uplifts and supports its most vulnerable members and those who care for them.

Chapter 1: A Crisis Ignored

The Elderly Crisis

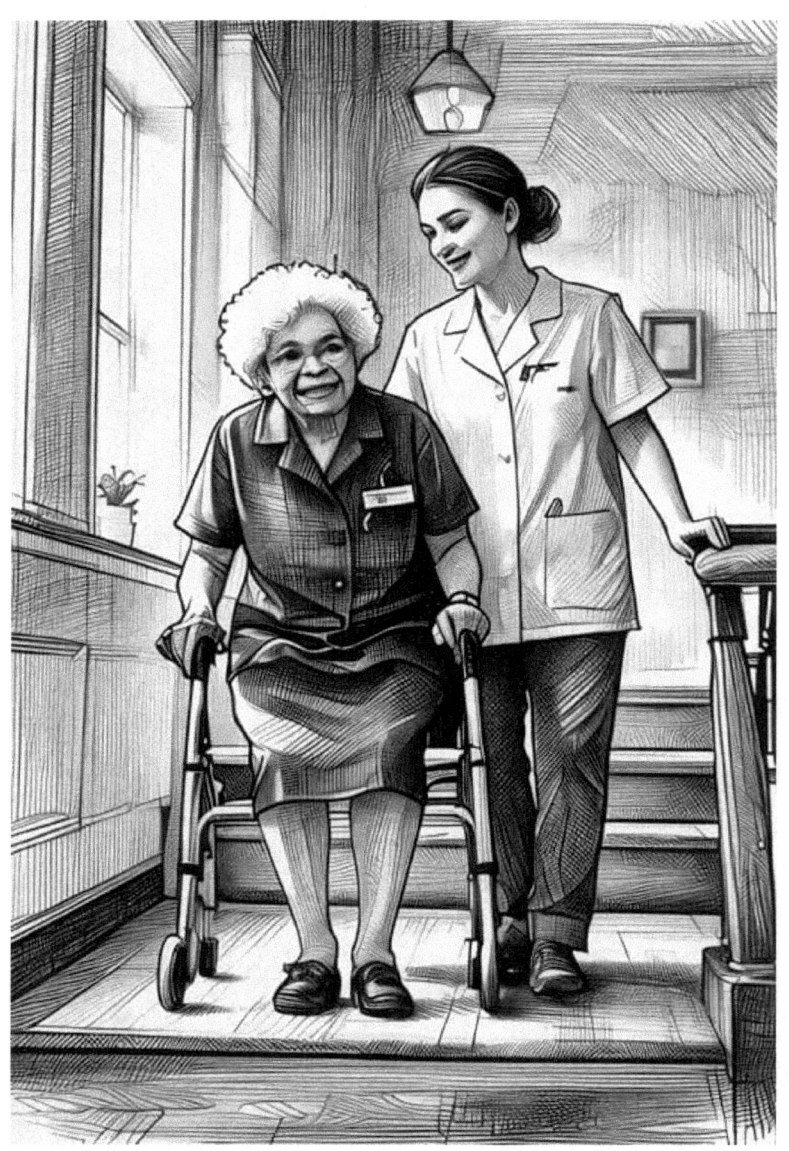

Chapter 2

The Breaking Point: When Caregiving Crushes Both Spirit and Body

The Human Cost of Elder Care: A Profound and Personal Journey

The "human cost" of elder care extends far beyond financial considerations, encompassing a profound and often unseen emotional, physical, and psychological toll on both the aging individuals themselves and the family members who undertake their care. This impact ripples through lives, altering relationships, reshaping daily routines, and demanding sacrifices that are often immeasurable. It's a journey I know intimately, having walked alongside my mother through her declining years. Let's delve into the multifaceted ways this "human cost" manifests.

For the Elderly: A Loss of Self and World

Loss of Independence:

As physical and cognitive decline sets in, the elderly often experience a gradual loss of independence. This can be incredibly difficult, leading to feelings of helplessness, frustration, and a diminished sense of self-worth. Simple tasks like bathing, dressing, and preparing meals may become challenging, impacting their daily routines and overall quality of life. My mum, a fiercely independent woman who had always been the pillar of strength for our family, struggled deeply with this loss. The frustration in her eyes when she couldn't manage everyday tasks was palpable, a stark reminder of the person she once was, and the limitations age had imposed. This need for independence is so important, especially for those who have lived their lives independently. It's a blow to their spirit, a challenge to their very identity.

Resolution:

- **Focus on Abilities:** Encourage seniors to focus on what they can do, rather than what they can't. Celebrate small victories and acknowledge their efforts.

- **Adaptive Tools:** Explore adaptive tools and assistive devices that can help seniors maintain some independence in daily tasks. Something as simple as a long-handled grabber for reaching items can make a huge difference.

- **Respectful Assistance:** Offer help with sensitivity and respect, avoiding language or actions that might undermine their dignity. Instead of taking over, offer assistance and guidance, allowing them to participate as much as possible.

Social Isolation and Loneliness:

Reduced mobility, declining health, and the loss of loved ones can lead to social isolation and loneliness. This can have a significant impact on mental and emotional well-being, increasing the risk of depression, anxiety, and even cognitive decline. Isolation due to declining health can even extend to the simple act of picking up the phone or making a call. Being left alone because people don't have time or make time to be around the elderly takes isolation to a deeper level. The TV being on, or music playing, doesn't make up for the feeling of being alone. Spending time and being present with someone is priceless, and many lessons can be learned, and wisdom gained from life's experiences. We need to put down our phones and spend time with one another; there we will find the hidden secrets of life that social media can never show us. Even though the tough times of taking care of my mum were in silence when she could no longer communicate, just being present taught me a lot of lessons, because I was able to use the time to reflect and think on the things she instilled in me and how I could use them to move forward and make me better.

Resolution:

- **Meaningful Connections:** Facilitate regular social interaction through visits, phone calls, video chats, or outings. Encourage participation in senior centers or community groups.

- **Intergenerational Programs:** Seek out programs that connect seniors with children or young adults for mutual benefit. These interactions can bring joy and a sense of purpose.

- **Pet Therapy:** Consider the possibility of pet ownership or regular visits from a therapy animal. The companionship and unconditional love of a pet can be incredibly beneficial.

  I recognize the invaluable role that companion animals play in the emotional well-being of seniors. My mother, throughout her life, found immense comfort and companionship in her beloved cats, from Shiny and Shady in her early years to Dusty and Stripes later on. These pets were a consistent source of joy and solace, providing unwavering emotional support through all stages of her life. Even as her memory began to decline, her bond with her feline companions remained strong, and she consistently recognized their presence. Remarkably, my mother outlived all her pets, yet in her final years, Stripes and Shady remained faithfully by her side until their peaceful passing, one under her bed and the other at her feet. When I returned home to care for my mother, my own cat, Silver, seamlessly integrated into her life, spending the last few months of my mum's life on her bed. This profound connection highlights how animals offer unconditional affection, reduce feelings of loneliness, and provide a sense of purpose and routine, all of which are critical for the emotional and psychological health of seniors. Their presence can significantly aid in coping with challenges, bringing immense comfort and stability during vulnerable times.

- **Technology for Connection:** Help seniors utilize technology for social connection, such as video calls, social media, or online games. Provide training and support to overcome any tech challenges.

Loss of Dignity:

Dependence on others for basic needs can sometimes lead to feelings of shame and a loss of dignity. Concerns about incontinence, frailty, and the potential for abuse can further erode self-esteem. This truly strips a person to the core, and in doing this for my mum, I remember seeing her face so frustrated yet so grateful to have someone she knew there to take care of her personal and private needs.

Resolution:

- **Respectful Care:** Provide personal care with sensitivity and respect, ensuring privacy and minimizing any feelings of embarrassment. Treat seniors with the same dignity and consideration you would want for yourself.

- **Choice and Control:** Whenever possible, offer seniors choices and control over their care. Allow them to make decisions about their daily routines, clothing, and personal preferences.

- **Positive Reinforcement:** Focus on seniors' strengths and abilities, offering positive reinforcement and encouragement. Help them maintain a sense of self-worth and value.

Fear of the Unknown:

Aging can bring a sense of uncertainty about the future, including declining health, loss of loved ones, and the potential need for long-term care. This fear can be overwhelming, leading to anxiety and distress.

Resolution:

- **Open Communication:** Encourage open and honest conversations about seniors' fears and concerns. Provide a safe space for them to express their anxieties without judgment.

- **Planning for the Future:** Involve seniors in discussions about their future care, including their preferences for healthcare, living arrangements, and end-of-life care. This can help alleviate anxiety and empower them to make informed choices.

- **Spiritual Support:** For seniors who are religious or spiritual, encourage them to draw on their faith for comfort and strength. Connect them with spiritual advisors or religious communities.

- **Focus on the Present:** Help seniors focus on the present moment, encouraging them to find joy and meaning in each day. Engage them in activities that bring them pleasure and a sense of purpose.

Beyond physical care and companionship, we made a conscious effort to engage my mother in a variety of activities tailored to her evolving capabilities and preferences. In her earlier years, she cherished reading and listening to her beloved gospel and reggae music. As Alzheimer's progressed, her interests shifted, and she found immense pleasure in looking at pictures in magazines and collecting stuffed toys. We consistently strived to keep her engaged and occupied through meaningful conversations and by reminiscing over photo albums. This commitment to active engagement is paramount for the elderly, as it provides cognitive stimulation, maintains a sense of purpose, and combats feelings of isolation. For family members and caregivers, facilitating these activities not only enriches the senior's life but also strengthens bonds and provides a sense of shared purpose. For the elderly themselves, sustained engagement can significantly enhance their quality of life, promote emotional well-being, and potentially slow cognitive decline, fostering a sense of dignity and continued connection to the world around them. For my mum, these moments of engagement, whether through music, pictures, or simply conversation, were invaluable, allowing her spirit to shine through even as her memory faded, a testament to her enduring vitality and joy.

By understanding these multifaceted challenges and implementing thoughtful solutions, we can create a more supportive and compassionate environment for our aging population, ensuring they age with dignity, respect, and connection. It's a journey we are all on, and by working together, we can make it a more meaningful and fulfilling experience for everyone.

The Caregiver's Burden: A Labor of Love and Sacrifice

Caregiving is a labor of love, a profound act of giving that often comes at a significant personal cost. It's a journey marked by physical strain, emotional challenges, financial pressures, and the constant negotiation of one's own needs against the needs of a loved one. This is a reality I know intimately, having dedicated six years to caring for my mother.

Physical Strain: The Body Bears Witness

Caregiving often involves physically demanding tasks, such as

Chapter 2: The Breaking Point

lifting, transferring, and assisting with personal care. This can lead to musculoskeletal injuries, chronic pain, and overall physical exhaustion. I can attest to this firsthand, having suffered neck and back injuries from the constant lifting and turning required in Mum's care. Yet, I remember telling myself, "As long as I can still move, I will carry on." While the long-term effects are undeniable, using assistive devices like braces and support apparatuses can make a significant difference, especially when you're the sole caregiver. It's crucial to be mentally strong and prioritize self-care, seeking help and utilizing available resources to alleviate the physical strain.

Resolution:

- **Proper Lifting Techniques:** Learn and practice proper lifting techniques to minimize the risk of injury. Utilize resources from healthcare professionals or online tutorials.

- **Assistive Equipment:** Invest in assistive equipment such as lifts, transfer belts, shower chairs, and adjustable beds to reduce physical strain.

- **Home Modifications:** Make necessary home modifications, such as grab bars, ramps, and widened doorways, to create a safer and more accessible environment.

- **Professional Help:** Don't hesitate to seek professional help from physical therapists or occupational therapists to develop strategies for safe and efficient caregiving.

- **Prioritize Self-Care:** Schedule regular exercise, stretching, and rest to maintain physical health and prevent burnout. Don't neglect your own medical needs.

Emotional Toll: A Rollercoaster of Feelings

Caregiving can be emotionally draining, with caregivers experiencing a wide range of feelings, including stress, anxiety, guilt, resentment, and grief. Witnessing the decline of a loved one can be incredibly challenging, and caregivers may experience anticipatory grief, mourning the loss of the person they once knew even while they are still alive. Seeing my mum deteriorate was heartbreaking, a constant reminder of the inevitable nature of aging and loss. Yet, I learned to find strength in knowing that we all age, and how we treat one another is a reflection of how we wish to be treated. It's essential to find mental fortitude and recognize that your loved one may be experiencing a form of second childhood, requiring patience and understanding. Not everyone is equipped to handle the emotional weight of caregiving. Counseling and support programs are vital resources for caregivers to process their emotions and develop coping mechanisms.

Resolution:

- **Seek Support:** Connect with support groups for caregivers, either in person or online. Sharing experiences with others who understand can be incredibly validating.
- **Therapy and Counseling:** Don't hesitate to seek professional help from a therapist or counselor specializing in caregiver stress and grief.
- **Prayer, Mindfulness and Meditation:** Pray daily. Practice mindfulness and meditation techniques to manage stress and cultivate inner peace.
- **Journaling:** Express your emotions and thoughts through journaling. This can be a cathartic way to process complex feelings.
- **Set Boundaries:** Learn to set healthy boundaries with family members and friends to protect your emotional well-being. It's okay to say "no" to

additional requests when you're feeling overwhelmed.

Financial Burden: The Cost of Caring

The costs associated with providing care can be significant, including medical expenses, home modifications, assistive equipment, and lost income due to reduced work hours or career changes. Caregiving can place a significant strain on personal finances. Preparing ahead of time can alleviate some of this burden. My mum's foresight in investing in long-term care insurance made a significant difference in our ability to provide her with the care she needed without financial strain. However, I also felt the financial impact of caregiving, having given up my own income for six years. While it taught me the valuable lesson that we can survive without luxuries, the financial realities of caregiving are undeniable.

Resolution:

Financial Planning: Develop a comprehensive financial plan that takes into account the potential costs of long-term care.

- **Explore Benefits:** Research and utilize available government programs, tax credits, and veterans' benefits to offset caregiving expenses.

- **Respite Care Assistance:** Seek out respite care programs that offer financial assistance or subsidies for caregivers.

- **Fundraising & Crowdfunding:** Consider utilizing online platforms to raise funds for specific caregiving needs, such as medical equipment or home modifications.

- **Legal and Financial Advice:** Consult with professionals specializing in elder law and financial planning to navigate the complexities of long-term care financing.

Social Isolation and Neglect of Self: The Vanishing Act

Caregivers often experience social isolation as their world shrinks to the confines of their loved one's needs. They may neglect their own social connections, hobbies, and personal interests, leading to feelings of loneliness and burnout. This isolation is often compounded by the lack of time and energy for self-care.

Resolution:

- **Schedule Breaks:** Prioritize scheduling regular breaks and time for yourself, even if it's just for a few hours each week. Utilize respite care services or ask family members for assistance.

- **Maintain Connections:** Make a conscious effort to stay connected with friends and family, even if it's just through phone calls or online interactions.

- **Pursue Hobbies:** Continue to engage in hobbies and activities that bring you joy and relaxation. Even short periods of engagement can make a difference.

- **Support Groups:** Connect with caregiver support groups to share experiences and build connections with others who understand.

- **Seek Professional Help:** If you're experiencing feelings of depression or burnout, don't hesitate to seek professional help from a therapist or counselor.

Caregiving is a challenging yet deeply rewarding experience. By acknowledging the burdens and implementing proactive strategies for support, we can empower caregivers to provide the best possible care while also prioritizing their own well-being. It's a journey that demands strength, resilience, and a willingness to ask for help. Remember, you are not alone.

Intergenerational Conflict: Navigating Family Dynamics in Elder Care

Caregiving responsibilities can place immense strain on family relationships, often leading to conflicts between siblings, spouses, and other family members. Resentment and guilt can arise, further complicating the caregiving experience. These conflicts can stem from disagreements about the level of care needed, financial contributions, living arrangements, or even differing opinions on medical treatment. It's crucial to remember that there's no single "right" way to approach elder care, and what works for one family may not work for another. Open communication, empathy, and a willingness to compromise are essential for navigating these challenging dynamics.

My own experience with caring for Mum alongside my brother, Steve, underscored the importance of teamwork and mutual respect. While we didn't always agree on every detail, we were committed to working together, prioritizing Mum's well-being above all else. This unity allowed us to present a united front, ensuring Mum felt secure and loved amidst the inevitable changes in her life.

Here are some common areas of conflict and potential resolutions:

Level of Care: One sibling may believe a parent needs full-time care in a facility, while another prefers in-home care.

Resolution:

- **Research and Education:** Gather information about different care options, including costs, benefits, and drawbacks. Consult with professionals like geriatricians or social workers.

- **Open Dialogue:** Hold family meetings to discuss each person's perspective, actively listening to concerns and rationale.

- **Compromise and Flexibility:** Be willing to compromise. Perhaps a trial period with in-home care, followed by reassessment, could be a solution.

- **Mediation:** If disagreements become entrenched,

consider seeking help from a professional mediator to facilitate constructive communication.

Financial Contributions: Disagreements about how much each family member can contribute financially can cause tension.

Resolution:

- **Transparency:** Create a shared spreadsheet or document outlining the costs of care and each person's financial capacity.

- **Fairness vs. Equality:** Recognize that equal contributions may not be feasible. Focus on what is fair and equitable, given individual circumstances.

- **Written Agreement:** Formalize financial agreements in writing to avoid misunderstandings or disputes later.

- **Professional Guidance:** Consult with a financial advisor or attorney specializing in elder law to explore options and ensure legal compliance.

Living Arrangements: Decisions about whether a parent should live with a family member or move to a care facility can be contentious.

Resolution:

- **Parents' Preferences:** Prioritize the parent's wishes whenever possible. Involve them in discussions and decision-making to the extent they are able.

- **Trial Periods:** Consider a trial period for co-residence to assess its feasibility for both the parent and the family member.

- **Neutral Territory:** If co-residence proves challenging, explore alternative living arrangements that offer a balance of independence and support.

- **Professional Assessment:** Seek guidance from a

social worker or geriatric care manager to assess the parents' needs and recommend appropriate living arrangements.

Medical Decisions: Differing opinions on medical treatment, end-of-life care, or the use of life-sustaining measures can lead to conflict.

Resolution:

- **Advance Directives:** Ensure the parent has completed advance directives, such as a living will and durable power of attorney for healthcare, clearly outlining their wishes.

- **Respecting Autonomy:** Honor the parents' autonomy and right to make their own medical decisions, even if family members disagree.

- **Open Communication with Medical Professionals:** Attend medical appointments together as a family to receive information and discuss treatment options with the healthcare team.

- **Ethics Consultation:** If disagreements arise regarding end-of-life care, consider seeking an ethics consultation through the healthcare provider.

Caregiving Responsibilities: One sibling may feel they are doing the lion's share of the work while others are less involved.

Resolution:

- **Task Breakdown:** Create a detailed list of caregiving tasks and assign responsibilities based on each family member's availability and capacity.

- **Regular Check-ins:** Schedule regular family meetings to discuss how the caregiving plan is working and make adjustments as needed.

- **Respite Support:** Offer respite care to the primary

caregiver to prevent burnout and ensure they have time for themselves.

- **Professional Assistance:** If family members are geographically dispersed or have limited availability, consider hiring a professional caregiver to supplement family efforts.

Remember, navigating intergenerational conflict in elder care requires empathy, patience, and a willingness to compromise. By prioritizing open communication, respecting individual perspectives, and focusing on the well-being of the aging parent, families can work together to provide the best possible care while preserving their own relationships. It's a journey best traveled together, supporting one another along the way.

In managing my mother's care, my brother Stephen and I, as her primary caregivers, maintained open communication and deeply respected each other's perspectives, collectively assuming all responsibilities. Our younger brother, Michael, despite his geographical distance and frequent work-related travel, remained an integral part of the important and urgent decision-making process. Michael was available by phone for crucial discussions concerning our mother's well-being if we needed him. This collaborative approach underscores the critical importance of assigning caregiving responsibilities based on individual family members' availability and capabilities, ensuring that support is both effective and sustainable. Through this period, Stephen and I gracefully embraced the challenges, committed to simply "getting it done" while steadfastly preserving our family harmony.

Chapter 2: The Breaking Point

The Elderly Crisis

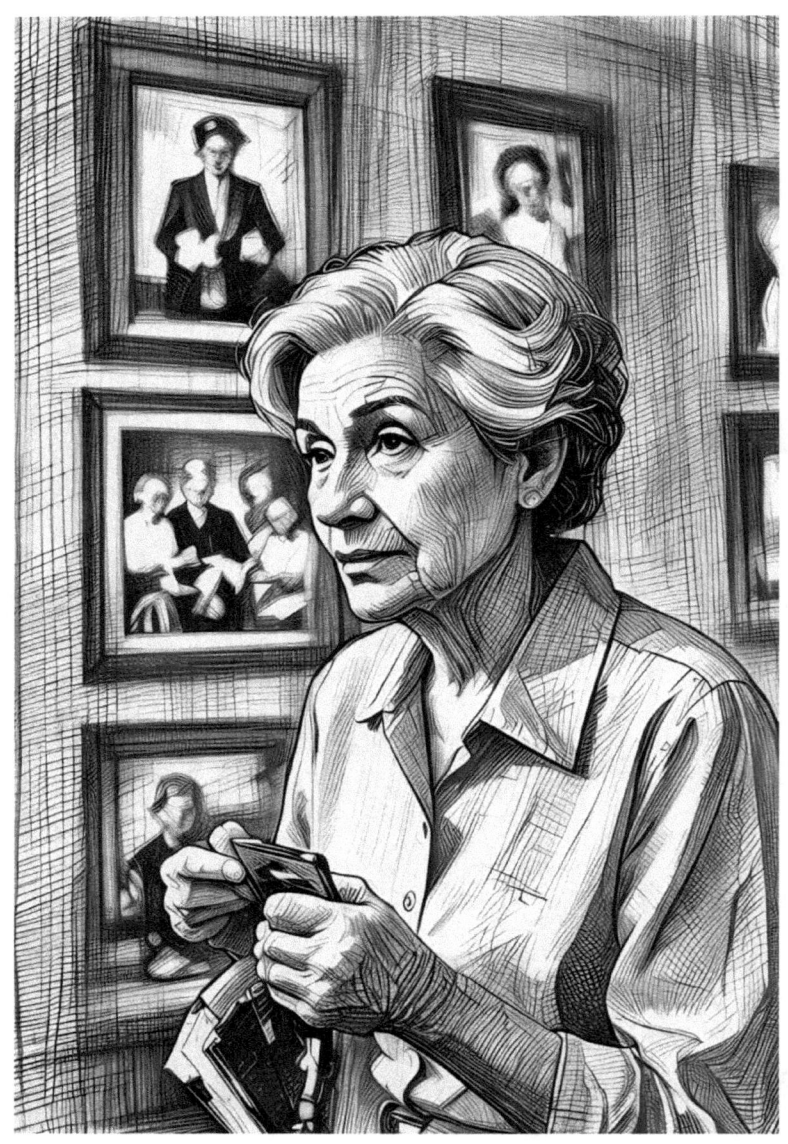

Chapter 3

Home Truths: The Difficulties Elders Face Within Families

Our Elders: A Tapestry of Love, Sacrifice, and Urgent Need

Our parents, our elders, represent a living history, a tapestry woven with threads of love, sacrifice, and unwavering devotion. They nurtured us, guided us, and shaped the individuals we are today. Yet, a heartbreaking crisis plagues our society: the neglect and abandonment of our aging loved ones.

It's a question that echoes in the hearts of many, a stark reminder of the shifting sands of societal values: Our parents sacrificed to take care of us as children, but most families don't and will not do the same when their parents get old. Why?

Cultural norms often play a significant role. In West Indian, Asian, African, and Spanish cultures, as I've observed, caring for elders within the family is often a deeply ingrained tradition. But even within these cultures, and certainly in others, the challenges of modern life can erode these traditions.

Having witnessed this firsthand alongside my longtime friend from England, Julie, I can attest to its profound impact. Julie has seen her own family fractured by disagreements concerning care, weighed down by financial pressures, or simply unable to dedicate the necessary time and resources for adequate support. Together, we've observed the resulting hardship on the elderly – the loneliness, the fear, the sense of abandonment.

It's easy to judge, to point fingers and assign blame. But the truth is, the reasons behind this crisis are complex. Some families struggle to balance the demands of work and childcare with the needs of an aging parent. Others may lack the space or resources to accommodate an elder in their home. Distance may also be a challenge if you live far apart, even in another country. And sadly, some may harbor resentment or unresolved conflicts that prevent them from offering care.

But, "Even if we were not offered the best of care growing up, now that we know better and can do better, shouldn't we give to our parents what they couldn't give us?" This is the crux of the matter. We have a moral obligation to care for those who once cared for us, to offer them the dignity, respect, and love they deserve in their twilight years.

It's important to remember that these are not universal experiences. Many families provide loving and supportive care to their elderly members. However, these are significant challenges that many families face, and addressing them requires open communication, empathy, and a focus on building strong and supportive family relationships throughout all stages of life. It was not easy for me and my brother, but we sacrificed our personal interests to provide for the needs of my mum, no matter how long it took. My friend Julie in the UK is the main caregiver for her mum, her support system comprises of care workers who visit twice daily to assist with her mum's daily needs. Many of her siblings live far away; others have health issues; some are simply not involved. Juggling all of this is a lot, but as friends, we were and are able to gain a greater understanding of the challenges and rewards of caregiving.

Here are some of the most important issues elderly individuals face within their families:

Chapter 3: Home Truths

Lack of Reciprocity: Many parents dedicate their lives to raising their children, often sacrificing their own needs and desires. However, when these parents reach old age, they may not receive the same level of care and support from their children. This can stem from various factors, including:

- **Shifting Family Dynamics:** Changing societal structures, such as increased geographic mobility and dual-income households, can make it more difficult for children to provide in-person care.

- **Generational Differences:** Differing expectations and communication styles between generations can create misunderstandings and resentment.

- **Burnout and Stress:** Caregiving responsibilities can be incredibly demanding, both physically and emotionally, leading to burnout and resentment among caregivers.

- **Financial Strain:** The costs associated with elder care can be substantial, and families may struggle to meet these financial obligations.

- **Lack of Awareness:** Some adult children may be unaware of the extent of their parents' needs or may underestimate the challenges of caregiving.

- **Unresolved Family Conflicts:** Past resentments or unresolved conflicts can resurface and hinder the ability of family members to work together effectively.

- **Lack of Support Systems:** Families may lack access to respite care, adult day care, or other support services that could ease the burden of caregiving.

- **Differing Values and Beliefs:** Family members may have different values or beliefs about elder care, leading to disagreements about the best course of action.

- **Emotional and Physical Distance:** Adult children who live far away from their parents may feel less connected to their needs and less able to provide hands-on care.

- **Family Conflict and Division:** Caregiving responsibilities can often lead to conflict among siblings, with disagreements arising over who should provide care, how care should be provided, and the division of financial burdens. These conflicts can strain family relationships and create lasting resentment.

- **Emotional Neglect and Abuse:** In some cases, elderly individuals may experience emotional neglect or abuse from family members, including: belittling or demeaning them, ignoring their needs or feelings, isolating them from friends or other family members, threatening or intimidating them, and verbal harassment or insults.

- **Financial Exploitation:** Misuse of the elderly person's finances.

- **Emotional Abuse:** Belittling, isolating, or controlling the elderly person.

- **Neglect:** Failing to provide necessities such as food, water, medication, and hygiene.

- **Lack of Communication and Planning:** Open and honest communication about future care needs is often lacking within families. This can lead to uncertainty, anxiety, and a lack of preparedness for the challenges of aging.

- **Intergenerational Guilt and Resentment:** Feelings of guilt and resentment can arise on both sides. Elderly parents may feel guilty for burdening their children. Children may feel guilty for not being able to provide the level of care they feel they should.

- **Elder Abuse:** Elder abuse is a serious problem that can take many forms, including physical, emotional, and financial abuse. It is often perpetrated by family members but can also occur in institutional settings.

- **Ageism:** Ageism is the stereotyping and discrimination against elderly individuals. It can manifest in many ways, from patronizing language to limited access to services and opportunities.

- **Isolation and Loneliness:** Elderly individuals are at increased risk for social isolation and loneliness, which can have a significant impact on their physical and mental health. This can be due to a number of factors, including the loss of loved ones, declining mobility, and lack of transportation.

- **Access to Technology:** Many elderly individuals are not comfortable with technology, which can make it difficult for them to stay connected with loved ones and access information and services online.

- **End-of-Life Care:** Planning for end-of-life care is important, but many families avoid these difficult conversations. This can lead to disagreements and conflict when the time comes.

It is important to remember that every family is different, and there is no one-size-fits-all solution to the challenges of elder care. However, by working together, communicating openly, and prioritizing the needs of their loved ones, families can find ways to provide the best possible care and support. It is also important to seek help from professionals, such as geriatric care managers, social workers, and financial advisors, when needed. They can provide valuable guidance and support to both elderly individuals and their families.

As my mum's journey neared its end, we knew we needed additional support. We embarked on a thorough search for home healthcare services, ultimately choosing ArchCare. It was a decision that brought immense comfort. The ArchCare nurses who visited twice a week were exceptional, providing diligent monitoring of vitals and invaluable assistance with other medical needs.

What truly set ArchCare apart was their ability to adapt and meet my mum's evolving needs. Whether it was adjusting visiting times, arranging necessary supplies, communicating seamlessly with her doctor, facilitating medical equipment, or collaborating on her overall care plan, they were consistently responsive and proactive. The level of support extended far beyond the remarkable nurses Gertrude and Maria. I received regular check-in calls from Manager Rosie Torres, whose care and dedication ensured my mum received the best possible attention. When Rosie wasn't available, Jeff and Evelyn stepped in seamlessly, providing the same level of commitment. Jeff, in particular, went above and beyond, working tirelessly with the doctors to coordinate my mum's medical supplies and equipment. In those challenging times, having a strong support system where you feel heard and valued, not just treated as a number, was truly a lifeline.

When Mum required end-of-life care, we entrusted her to Calvary Hospice. Manager Tierny Simmons and nurse Maggie Heenan expertly navigated the complexities of this transition with compassion and grace. End-of-life care is undeniably the most challenging phase, as the inevitable outcome becomes clear. Maggie's extensive experience with Calvary made her an ideal caregiver for my mum, especially given that my mum was a nurse herself, setting a high standard for her care. On the morning of my mum's passing, Manager Tierny paid a final tribute by personally coming to pronounce her death and saluting a fellow nurse.

To ArchCare and Calvary Hospice, and to Rosie Torres, Jeffrey Golman, Evelyn Morales, Tierny Simmons, and Maggie Heenan: words cannot fully express the depth of our gratitude. Your expertise, compassion, and unwavering support made an incredibly difficult journey more bearable. You provided not only exceptional care for my mum but also invaluable support for our family. Thank you, sincerely.

The Nursing Home Dilemma: Last Resort or Best Option?

Too often, nursing homes are seen as the easy solution, a way to absolve ourselves of responsibility. But I ask you, "Would you want to be kept in a nursing home?" For many elderly individuals, the answer is a resounding no.

Nursing homes can offer valuable services, particularly for those with complex medical needs. They provide 24-hour care, access to medical professionals, and a structured environment. But they also come with drawbacks.

- **Loss of Familiarity:** Moving to a nursing home means leaving behind a lifetime of memories, familiar surroundings, and cherished possessions. This can be disorienting and emotionally distressing for elders, exacerbating feelings of loss and confusion.

- **Isolation and Loneliness:** Despite the presence of other residents, many elderly individuals in nursing homes experience profound loneliness. They may miss the close relationships with family and friends, the comfort of familiar routines, and the sense of belonging.

- **Decline in Health:** Studies have shown that elderly individuals in nursing homes often experience a decline in both physical and cognitive health. This may be due to the stress of adapting to a new environment, reduced social interaction, or a lack of personalized care.

However, it's also important to acknowledge that nursing homes can be a necessary option for some families. When a loved one requires specialized medical care that cannot be

The Elderly Crisis

provided at home, or when the burden of caregiving becomes unsustainable for family members, a nursing home can offer a safe and supportive environment.

Chapter 3: Home Truths

The Elderly Crisis

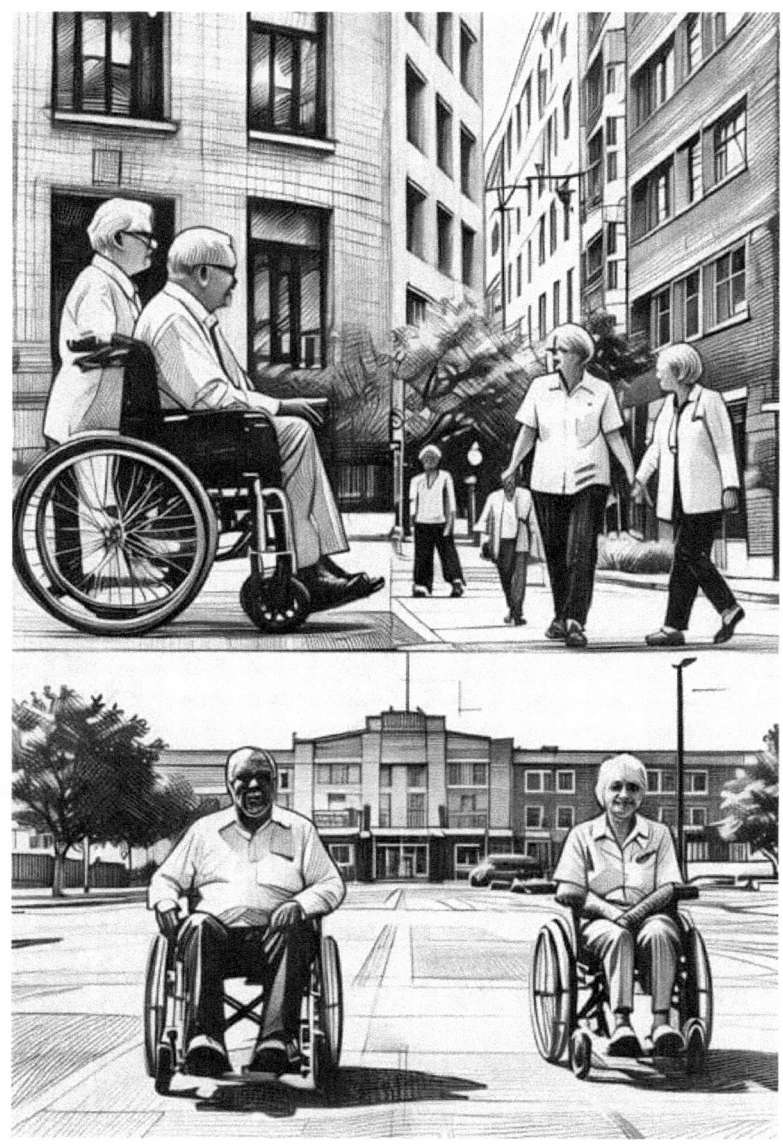

Chapter 4

Systems That Fail: When Nations and the World Abandon Their Elders

Let's Examine the Failures of our Nationwide and Global Systems:

The failures and shortcomings of our national and global systems are numerous and complex, placing a great strain on millennials. While it's true that more attention is often paid to the up-and-coming younger generation, millennials are facing significant challenges that demand attention. Here are some of the most critical issues, highlighting both national and global dimensions and drawing parallels between countries and states:

1. National Level

Inequality: This pervasive issue manifests in various forms, mirroring global trends.

- **Economic Inequality:** The chasm between the wealthy and the impoverished continues to expand, mirroring the global wealth gap. This disparity fuels social and economic instability, evident in limited access to quality education, healthcare, affordable housing, and equitable opportunities. Just as certain countries dominate global wealth, within nations, specific regions or demographics often experience disproportionate economic disadvantage.
- **Racial and Ethnic Inequality:** Systemic racism remains deeply entrenched, echoing historical patterns of discrimination seen across the globe. This results in

disparities in outcomes for people of color in areas like criminal justice (with parallels to discriminatory practices in various countries), employment (similar to global disparities in labor opportunities), and housing (reflecting global patterns of segregation and unequal access to resources).

- **Gender Inequality:** Women continue to encounter discrimination in the workplace, underrepresentation in leadership roles, and persistent pay gaps, mirroring global struggles for gender equality. Like many nations, individual states or regions within a country may have more pronounced gender disparities due to cultural or legal factors.

Political Polarization: Extreme political division leads to governmental gridlock, hindering progress on crucial issues such as climate change, healthcare, and infrastructure, mirroring the challenges of international cooperation on global issues. This erosion of trust in institutions and the fueling of social unrest are also seen in various forms across the globe.

Environmental Degradation: Many nations, similar to the global community, fail to adequately address environmental challenges like climate change, pollution, and resource depletion. The severe consequences for public health, biodiversity, and long-term sustainability are felt both locally and globally. Just as some nations are more vulnerable to climate change, certain states or regions within a country may face greater environmental risks.

Mass Incarceration: The United States' high incarceration rate, with its disproportionate impact on Black and Brown communities, reflects a global problem of over-incarceration and systemic biases within justice systems. Like international disparities in justice, specific states or regions within the US have significantly higher rates of incarceration for minority populations.

Access to Healthcare: Limited access to affordable and quality healthcare, plagued by high costs, administrative burdens, and disparities based on income and location, is a challenge faced by many nations. Similar to global inequalities in healthcare access, within a country, certain states or regions may have greater challenges in providing adequate healthcare.

2. Global Level

Climate Change: The global community's inadequate response to climate change, despite agreements like the Paris Agreement, mirrors the challenges nations face in implementing effective climate policies. The devastating consequences, including extreme weather, rising sea levels, and biodiversity loss, are shared globally, but also disproportionately affect vulnerable populations within and across nations.

Global Inequality: The widening gap between the richest and poorest countries, with a small number controlling a disproportionate share of global wealth, is mirrored by economic inequality within nations. This fuels poverty, conflict, and instability globally, and similar patterns of disparity and unrest can be observed within individual countries.

Geopolitical Tensions: Rising geopolitical tensions, often fueled by competition for resources, ideological differences, and historical grievances, hinder international cooperation on shared challenges. These tensions are also reflected within nations, where regional or political divisions can create significant obstacles to progress.

Having been born and raised in the UK and now living in the United States, I've compared the services for the elderly in both countries. This comparison highlights how the value placed on the elderly is dependent on geographical location.

Comparing British and American Systems for the Elderly:

Who Provides Better Services? Both the UK and the US face similar challenges regarding aging populations, but their approaches to elder care differ significantly. Neither system is perfect; each has strengths and weaknesses. Directly declaring one "better" is difficult, as individual needs and experiences vary greatly.

However, we can compare key aspects:

Healthcare:

- **UK:** The National Health Service (NHS) provides universal healthcare, largely funded through taxation. This means most services, including hospital care, doctor's visits, and some home care, are free at the point of use for seniors. However, waiting lists for certain procedures and social care services can be a challenge.

- **US:** Healthcare is a complex mix of private insurance, government programs like Medicare (for those 65+), and Medicaid (for low-income individuals). Medicare doesn't cover everything (e.g., long-term care, dental, vision), and out-of-pocket costs can be substantial. Access to quality care is often tied to income and insurance coverage.

Long-Term Care:

- **UK:** The system is means-tested, meaning eligibility for government-funded long-term care depends on assets and income. Those with significant needs and limited resources may receive assistance, but funding cuts have impacted availability and quality. Many rely on unpaid family caregivers.

- **US:** Long-term care is primarily a private responsibility. Medicaid covers some costs for those who qualify (low-income and assets), but the eligibility requirements are strict. Long-term care insurance is an option for some, but premiums can be high. Many

Chapter 4: Systems That Fail

Americans face significant out-of-pocket expenses or rely on family support.

Social Care:

- **UK:** Local councils provide social care services, including home care, meals on wheels, and day centers, but funding reductions have impacted availability and quality. Eligibility criteria are often stringent.

- **US:** A patchwork of government programs (often at the state level) and non-profit organizations offer some social services, but access varies widely. Many seniors rely on family, friends, or paid help.

Financial Support:

- **UK:** The state pension provides a basic income for retirees and means-tested benefits offer additional support for those with low incomes.

- **US:** Social Security provides a basic retirement income for most workers, but the amount depends on earnings history. Supplemental Security Income (SSI) is available for low-income seniors and disabled individuals.

Key Differences & Considerations:

- **Universal vs. Targeted:** The UK emphasizes universal access to healthcare, while the US system is more fragmented and tied to income/insurance.

- **Funding:** The UK system is primarily tax-funded, while the US relies on a mix of public and private funding.

- **Access:** The UK offers more equitable access to basic healthcare, but waiting lists can be a problem. The US offers greater choice and potentially faster access for those with good insurance, but access is unequal.

- **Long-Term Care:** Both countries face challenges in providing affordable and accessible long-term care. The UK system is more reliant on means-testing, while the US system is more reliant on private resources.

Who Provides Better Services?

It's not a simple answer. The UK system may offer better access to basic healthcare and financial support for low-income seniors. However, the US system may provide more choice and potentially faster access to specialized care for those with good insurance. Both systems struggle with long-term care, and both rely heavily on unpaid family caregivers.

Ultimately, the "better" system depends on the individual's needs and circumstances. Both countries need to address the challenges of aging populations by improving access to affordable long-term care, strengthening social care services, and providing greater support for family caregivers.

I found the healthcare system in the US to be more advantageous for my mother. Because she had excellent coverage and insurance, she had immediate access to medical care and was able to select her healthcare providers and physicians. If a doctor or provider wasn't meeting her needs, we could easily find another; we had the power and control to make changes. In contrast, the UK system offers less choice, as it controls and dictates overall care, and the wait lists can create significant disadvantages.

Chapter 4: Systems That Fail

The Elderly Crisis

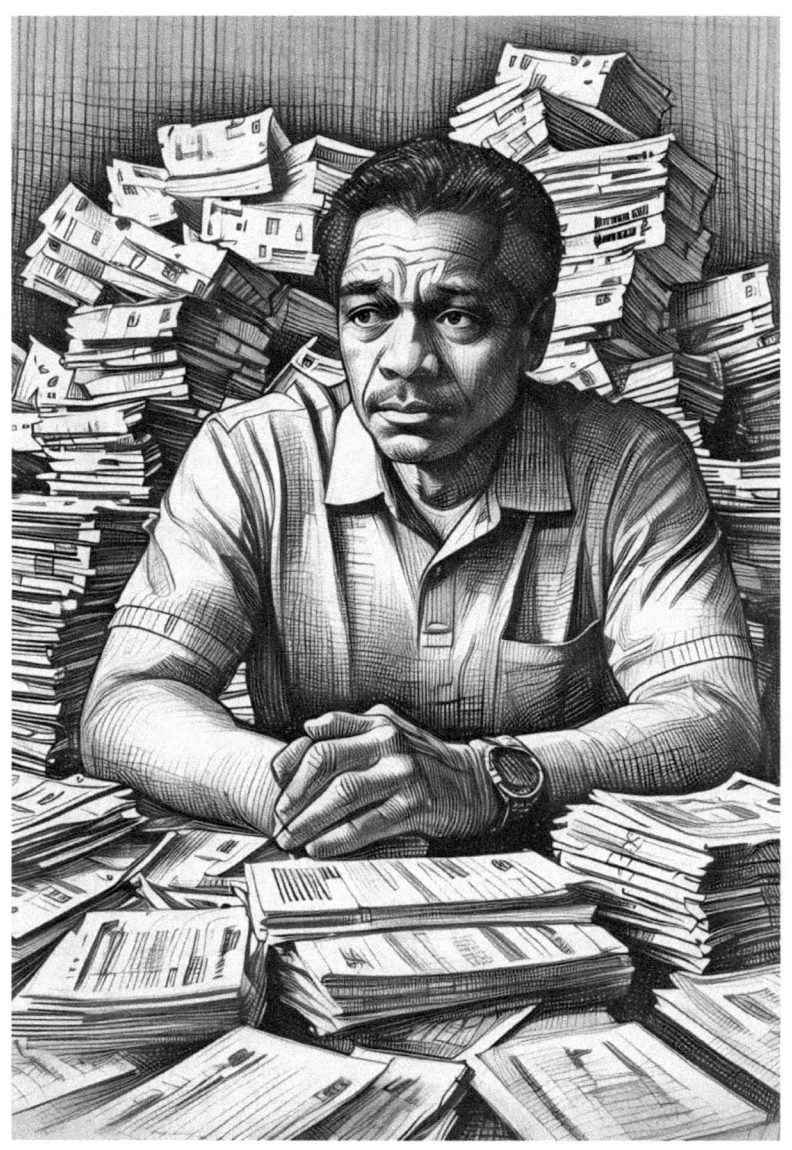

Chapter 5

The Price of Dignity: How Finances Shatter the Dream of a Secure Old Age

The Crushing Cost of Caring: A Personal and Societal Crisis

The financial burdens associated with long-term care for the elderly are staggering and continue to escalate, creating a perfect storm of challenges for individuals, families, and our healthcare system. It's a reality I know intimately, having witnessed firsthand the toll it takes. Educating families about preparing for their senior years is paramount. Additional policies and long-term investments are crucial. And planning for end-of-life expenses is not just practical, it's an act of love. I discovered paperwork from ten years ago that Mum hadn't followed up on regarding a burial plot. The price she had been quoted in 2015, around $5,000, had ballooned to $20,000 a decade later. It's a stark example of how inflation erodes our ability to plan for these inevitable costs. Many people set aside money for funeral expenses, but securing specific items in advance can significantly lessen the financial burden later.

Here's a breakdown of the financial realities of long-term care:

High and Rising Costs:
- **Nursing Homes:** The cost of nursing home care is astronomical, with the average annual cost exceeding $100,000 in many areas. This can quickly deplete a lifetime of savings.

- **Assisted Living:** While generally less expensive than nursing homes, assisted living facilities still represent a substantial financial commitment, often ranging from $3,000 to $10,000 per month.
- **Home Care:** Home care services, including home health aides, can be surprisingly expensive, especially for individuals requiring extensive assistance. Even a few hours of help per week can add up significantly.

Limited Coverage:

- **Medicare:** Medicare, the federal health insurance program for those 65 and older, primarily covers short-term skilled nursing care following a hospital stay. It does not cover the ongoing costs of long-term care.
- **Medicaid:** Medicaid, a joint federal and state program providing healthcare for low-income individuals, does cover some long-term care costs. However, eligibility is typically dependent on depleting the majority of one's assets, making it a "safety net" rather than a reliable source of long-term care financing for most middle-class individuals.
- **Long-Term Care Insurance:** Long-term care insurance is designed to help cover these costs, but it's not a silver bullet. Premiums can be prohibitively expensive, especially for those with pre-existing health conditions, and policies may have limitations or caps on coverage.

Inflationary Pressures:

The cost of long-term care is increasing at a rate far outpacing general inflation, making it increasingly challenging for individuals and families to afford these essential services. This is fueled by several factors:

- **Aging Population:** As the population ages, the

demand for long-term care services increases, driving up costs.

- **Increased Demand for Services:** Advances in medical technology mean people are living longer, often requiring care for extended periods.
- **Rising Healthcare Costs:** The overall cost of healthcare continues to rise, impacting all aspects of care, including long-term care.

Lack of Financial Preparedness:

Many individuals and families are woefully unprepared for the financial realities of long-term care. They may:

- **Underestimate Costs:** Not fully grasp the sheer magnitude of long-term care expenses.
- **Lack Adequate Savings:** Fail to save sufficiently for retirement, leaving little to cover potential long-term care needs.
- **Delay Planning:** Put off planning for long-term care, missing opportunities to explore insurance options or other financial strategies.

Impact on Family Finances:

The financial burden of long-term care can be devastating for families, leading to:

- **Depleted Savings:** Wipe out a lifetime of savings.
- **Forced Sale of Assets:** Necessitate selling homes, cars, or other assets to pay for care.
- **Bankruptcy:** In some cases, even lead to bankruptcy.

Caregivers also experience significant financial strain due to:

- **Lost Income:** Reduced work hours or leaving the workforce entirely to provide care.
- **Increased Expenses:** Paying for medications, supplies, or other care-related costs.

- **Reduced Earning Potential:** Impact on career trajectory due to caregiving responsibilities.

Caring for Mum full-time meant sacrificing not only my time but also my financial stability. Without an income, and with her unable to qualify for support, I had to stretch limited savings and past investments to cover my personal needs. It was a constant balancing act, prioritizing her well-being above my own, often going without myself. This sacrifice was deeply personal and, I know, not feasible for everyone. My circumstances were unique; I had no children, no partner, nor other dependents relying on me. Through this experience, I learned a powerful lesson: we truly don't need a lot in life. Material possessions provide comfort, perhaps, but they are not true necessities. Now that Mum has passed, I carry this wisdom forward. I'm committed to managing my finances more intentionally, focusing on investments and the things in life that are truly essential. More importantly, I want to dedicate my time and resources to helping others.

The Expanding Need:

The continued increase in demand for long-term care is driven by two key factors:

- **A Larger Aging Population:** The number of elderly individuals requiring care is steadily rising.

- **Increased Life Expectancy:** People are living longer, often with chronic conditions that necessitate extended care.

This presents a complex challenge with no easy solutions. However, by acknowledging the financial realities, planning ahead, and advocating for policy changes that support both individuals and families, we can strive to lessen this burden and ensure our elders receive the dignified care they deserve.

In conclusion, supporting caregivers and seniors through policy changes is not only compassionate but also a sound economic and social investment. By alleviating the financial

Chapter 5: The Price of Dignity

strain of caregiving, we can ensure our loved ones receive the care they need while also protecting the well-being of caregivers and families. This will create a more just and sustainable system that values the contributions of caregivers and upholds the dignity of our aging population.

The Elderly Crisis

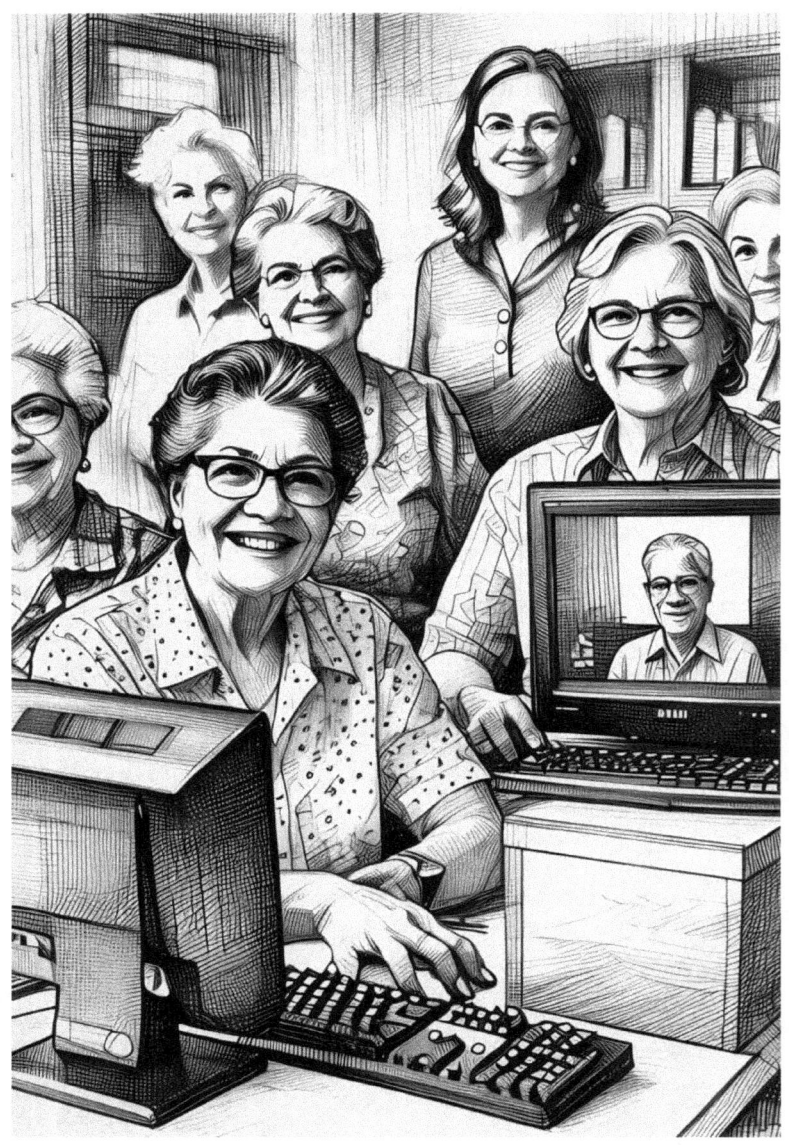

Chapter 6

A Call to Action: Reclaiming Humanity for Our Forgotten Generation

Combating Elder Neglect: A Multifaceted Approach

Elder neglect is a pervasive societal issue with devastating consequences for our aging population. It takes many forms, ranging from the deprivation of basic necessities like food, water, and medication to emotional abandonment and social isolation. Often, it arises from a complex combination of factors affecting both the elderly individual and their caregivers. Effective solutions require a comprehensive and multifaceted approach that addresses these root causes, provides robust support systems, and recognizes that families, while often the primary source of care, can also be the source of neglect. Therefore, we must broaden our focus to include community support networks, neighbors, and the healthcare system in our efforts to protect vulnerable seniors.

Here are some innovative and impactful strategies to combat elder neglect:

Strengthening Community Support Networks:

- **Expanded Neighborhood Watch Programs:** While the concept of neighborhood watch programs extending to include regular check-ins on elderly residents is laudable, its practicality varies greatly depending on the specific neighborhood context. In theory, volunteers can offer companionship, identify potential needs, and report concerns to relevant authorities, fostering a sense of community responsibility and providing a safety net for vulnerable seniors. However, several challenges must be considered. Safety can be a significant concern, both for the elderly residents themselves and the volunteers participating in the watch. In some neighborhoods, fear of crime or distrust within the community may hinder participation and effectiveness. Furthermore, the safety of elderly individuals can be compromised if volunteers are not properly vetted or trained to recognize signs of abuse or neglect. Therefore, implementing such programs requires careful planning, including thorough background checks for volunteers, comprehensive training on elder care and safety protocols, and establishing clear communication channels with law enforcement and social services.

Alternative strategies, particularly for densely populated urban areas where traditional neighborhood watch models may be less feasible, could include:

- **Community Partnerships with Local Businesses:** Establishing relationships with local businesses, such as pharmacies, grocery stores, and restaurants, to train employees to recognize signs of elder neglect or distress among their elderly customers.

- **Targeted Outreach Programs:** Focusing on reaching out to elderly individuals through community centers, senior centers, and religious institutions, providing information about available resources and support services.

- **Utilizing Technology:** Exploring the use of technology, such as community alert systems or neighborhood social media groups, to disseminate information and facilitate communication among residents regarding the well-being of elderly neighbors.

In contrast, traditional neighborhood watch models may be more effective in suburban and rural areas characterized by stronger community cohesion and lower crime rates. Even in these areas, however, supplementing neighborhood watch programs with security measures such as security cameras and alarm systems can enhance safety and provide an additional layer of protection for elderly residents. Ultimately, a tailored approach that considers the specific needs and characteristics of each community is crucial for successfully leveraging community support networks to prevent elder neglect.

Community Meals and Centers:

Community meals and senior centers play a crucial role in combating social isolation, a significant risk factor for elder neglect. By providing opportunities for seniors to connect with others through shared meals, social activities, and educational programs, these initiatives foster a sense of belonging and reduce loneliness. Beyond social interaction, these centers can serve as vital hubs for information and resources, linking seniors with essential services such as transportation assistance, healthcare referrals, and legal aid. Regular community meals also offer a valuable opportunity to informally monitor seniors' well-being, including their dietary intake and overall health. Observing changes in appetite or physical appearance can provide early warning signs of potential neglect or health issues, allowing for timely intervention.

Intergenerational Programs:

Intergenerational programs offer a unique and mutually beneficial approach to addressing elder neglect. By bridging the gap between generations through structured programs that encourage interaction and mutual support, these initiatives foster empathy and understanding while providing practical assistance to seniors. Younger individuals can assist with errands, technology, home maintenance, and companionship, reducing isolation and providing seniors with a sense of purpose. Local schools can play a vital role in these programs, offering students opportunities for community engagement through internships, paid work programs, or extra credit for off-site outreach. Carefully designed programs can even serve as a training ground, introducing young people to careers in healthcare or social services and preparing them to become future caregivers or advocates for the elderly.

Senior Companion Programs:

Senior companion programs, which pair volunteers with seniors at high risk of isolation or neglect, provide invaluable emotional support and assistance with daily tasks. These regular visits can significantly improve seniors' quality of life, reducing feelings of loneliness and providing a vital link to the outside world. Companions can offer a listening ear, engage seniors in stimulating activities, and help them access necessary resources. However, the time commitment required for effective companionship can be a challenge for volunteers. Elderly individuals often require extensive time, patience, and understanding, extending far beyond a few hours a week. Recruiting dedicated volunteers and providing them with adequate training and support are essential for the success of these programs. Furthermore, it's crucial to recognize that companionship alone may not be sufficient for seniors with complex needs. Coordinating companion services with other support systems, such as home healthcare or personal care assistance, is often necessary to ensure comprehensive care.

Enhancing Caregiver Support: A Vital Component in Elder Care

Caregivers are the unsung heroes of elder care, dedicating their time, energy, and often their personal resources to providing essential support to their loved ones. However, the demands of caregiving can be overwhelming, leading to burnout, financial strain, and social isolation. Robust support systems for caregivers are not just a matter of compassion;

Chapter 6: A Call to Action

they are crucial for ensuring quality care for seniors and preventing elder neglect.

Here are some key strategies to enhance caregiver support:

Respite Care Programs:

Respite care, offering temporary relief for caregivers, is essential for preventing burnout and allowing caregivers to recharge. Accessible and affordable respite options are crucial, ranging from a few hours a week to extended overnight stays, with some European countries even offering programs extending to several days or a week, recognizing the long-term nature of caregiving needs. Expanding respite care options could include increased government funding to support respite care services and make them more affordable, the development of mobile respite care teams that can provide in-home support, partnerships with community organizations and volunteers to offer low-cost or free respite options, tax credits or subsidies for families who utilize respite care services, the expansion of adult day care programs to provide social engagement and care for elders, offering respite for daytime caregivers, the creation of short-term stay programs in assisted living or nursing facilities specifically for respite purposes, awareness campaigns to inform caregivers about available respite resources and encourage their utilization, training and support for family members who can provide respite care for each other, and technology-based solutions to connect caregivers with available respite providers.

Flexible Respite Models:

Offer a variety of respite options, including in-home care, adult day care centers, short-term residential stays, and peer support programs. This allows caregivers to choose options that best fit their needs and their loved one's preferences.

Subsidized Respite Care:

Provide financial assistance or subsidies to make respite care more affordable, removing financial barriers that prevent caregivers from accessing this vital support.

Respite Care Navigation Services:

Establish centralized resources to help caregivers navigate the complex landscape of respite care options, including eligibility requirements, program availability, and funding assistance.

Caregiver Support Groups: Support groups provide a safe and supportive space for caregivers to share experiences, receive emotional support, and learn coping strategies. Connecting with others who understand the challenges of caregiving can reduce feelings of isolation and being overwhelmed. However, traditional in-person support groups can be difficult for busy caregivers to attend. To enhance accessibility:

- **Online Support Groups:** Offer virtual support groups via video conferencing or online forums, allowing caregivers to participate from the comfort of their homes and at times that are convenient for them.

- **Specialized Support Groups:** Create support groups tailored to specific caregiving challenges, such as caring for someone with dementia, managing challenging behaviors, or coping with grief and loss.

- **Peer-to-Peer Support Programs:** Develop programs that connect experienced caregivers with newer caregivers to provide mentorship and guidance.

Caregiver Education and Training:

Equipping caregivers with the knowledge and skills they need to provide quality care is essential. This includes training on:

- **Elder Care Techniques:** Safe lifting and transferring techniques, personal care assistance, medication management, and recognizing signs of illness or distress.

- **Stress Management:** Coping mechanisms for managing stress, setting boundaries, and prioritizing self-care.
- **Legal and Financial Issues:** Information about legal rights, financial planning, and accessing resources for seniors.
- **Recognizing and Reporting Abuse and Neglect:** Training on identifying signs of elder abuse and neglect, and procedures for reporting concerns to the appropriate authorities.

Financial Assistance and Tax Credits:

Recognize the significant financial burden of caregiving by providing financial assistance, tax credits, or subsidies to help cover expenses related to care. This could include:

- **Direct Financial Assistance:** Provide stipends or grants to caregivers to help offset the costs of caregiving expenses.
- **Tax Credits and Deductions:** Offer tax credits or deductions for eligible caregiving expenses, such as medical costs, home modifications, and respite care.
- **Paid Family Leave:** Implement paid family leave policies that allow employees to take time off from work to care for a family member without jeopardizing their income or job security.

By implementing these comprehensive strategies, we can create a more supportive environment for caregivers, ensuring they have the resources and support they need to provide quality care while also protecting their own well-being. Investing in caregiver support is an investment in the well-being of our seniors and the strength of our communities.

Improving Technology and Accessibility for Elder Care:

A Balanced Approach

Technology offers tremendous potential to enhance the lives of seniors and support their caregivers. However, it's crucial to acknowledge that a "one-size-fits-all" approach is not effective. Accessibility, user-friendliness, and individual preferences must be carefully considered to ensure technology truly benefits older adults.

Here's a breakdown of key areas and considerations:

Telehealth Services:

Expanding access to telehealth services can revolutionize elder care, particularly for those in rural areas or with mobility limitations. Remote monitoring of vital signs, video consultations with healthcare professionals, and virtual therapy sessions can improve access to care, reduce travel burdens, and facilitate timely medical interventions.

- **Pros:** Increased access to specialists, reduced healthcare costs, improved medication adherence through remote monitoring, and greater convenience for both seniors and caregivers.

- **Cons:** Requires reliable internet access and digital literacy, potential privacy concerns, limitations in physical examinations, and challenges in addressing complex medical needs remotely. Furthermore, as my mum's experience with Alzheimer's highlighted, cognitive decline can significantly hinder the effective use of telehealth, particularly when communication and memory are compromised. In such cases, the human element of in-person care remains essential.

Smart Home Technologies:

Smart home devices can assist with daily living activities, promoting independence and safety for seniors. Examples include medication reminders, fall detection systems, remote monitoring by family members, and smart home devices that can be controlled remotely (e.g., lights, thermostat, appliances).

- **Pros:** Enhanced safety through fall detection and emergency alerts, improved medication adherence, increased independence in managing daily tasks, and greater peace of mind for family members.

- **Cons:** High upfront costs for devices and installation, potential learning curve for seniors unfamiliar with technology, privacy concerns related to data collection, and reliance on technology that can malfunction or be hacked. Moreover, as with telehealth, cognitive decline can limit the effective use of smart home technologies. For instance, someone with dementia may struggle to remember how to use medication reminders or may become confused by voice-activated devices. A high level of independence and cognitive function is often necessary for successful adoption.

Accessible Technology Training:

Providing training and support to ensure that technology is accessible and user-friendly for older adults is crucial. This includes training on smartphones, tablets, computers, and online resources, empowering seniors to stay connected and access information independently.

- **Pros:** Increased digital literacy, reduced social isolation through online communication, enhanced access to information and resources, and greater independence in managing daily tasks.

- **Cons:** Many seniors are resistant to adopting new technologies, citing concerns about complexity, cost, and privacy. Age-related physical limitations, such as vision or hearing loss, can also pose challenges. Furthermore, as people age, there can be a natural inclination to do less, not more, making the adoption of new, potentially challenging technologies less appealing. Effective training programs must be patient, personalized, and tailored to the specific needs and learning styles of older adults. Motivation and ongoing support are key to overcoming resistance and fostering digital literacy.

Moving Forward:

Technology holds immense promise for improving the lives of seniors and supporting their caregivers. However, it's essential to approach technology adoption with a balanced perspective, acknowledging both the potential benefits and the inherent challenges. Prioritizing accessibility, providing comprehensive training, and addressing individual needs and preferences are crucial for ensuring that technology empowers, rather than overwhelms, older adults. Furthermore, it's vital to recognize that technology should complement, not replace, the human element of care.

Compassionate, in-person support remains essential for addressing the complex needs of our aging population.

Strengthening Legal and Regulatory Frameworks to Protect Elders:

Robust legal and regulatory frameworks are essential to prevent elder abuse and neglect, holding perpetrators accountable and ensuring justice for victims. Increased funding for Adult Protective Services (APS) is paramount. APS agencies must be adequately funded and staffed with trained professionals to promptly and effectively investigate reports of abuse, neglect, and exploitation. This includes providing resources for victim support, legal assistance, and protective services, such as temporary guardianship or relocation to a safe environment. Enhanced penalties for elder abuse are crucial to deter these crimes and signal a clear societal intolerance for such actions. Stricter penalties must be enforced for individuals who abuse, neglect, or exploit older adults, whether family members, caregivers, or professionals. Mandatory reporting requirements and comprehensive training for professionals who interact with older adults are vital. Healthcare providers, social workers, financial advisors, and other professionals must be trained to recognize the subtle signs of abuse and neglect, understand their legal obligations to report suspected cases, and follow proper reporting procedures. This training should also cover cultural sensitivities and ethical considerations related to elder care.

Promoting Open Communication and Planning for Elder Care:

Open communication and proactive planning within families are crucial for ensuring seniors' needs are met and their wishes are respected. Advance care planning, which encourages open and honest conversations about future care needs, including end-of-life care decisions, is essential. This involves discussing preferences for medical treatment, living arrangements, financial matters, and other critical aspects of care, ensuring that the elderly individual's voice is heard, and their autonomy is honored. Legal and financial planning assistance is vital for older adults. Providing resources and assistance with estate planning, financial planning, and the appointment of a trusted individual to manage affairs in case of incapacity can protect seniors from financial exploitation and ensure their assets are managed according to their wishes. This assistance should be accessible regardless of income level.

Addressing Social Determinants of Health to Reduce Elder Neglect:

Social determinants of health, such as poverty, inequality, lack of access to affordable housing, and inadequate transportation, significantly impact the risk of elder neglect. Reducing poverty and inequality through social programs, living wage initiatives, and access to education and employment opportunities can improve the overall well-being of seniors and their families, reducing the stressors that can contribute to neglect. Improving access to affordable housing and transportation is also critical. Ensuring that older adults have access to safe, affordable housing options that meet their needs, including accessible design and proximity to essential services, promotes independence and reduces the risk of isolation. Improved transportation options for seniors who no longer drive, such as public transportation, ride-sharing programs, or volunteer driver services, enable them to maintain social connections, access healthcare appointments, and participate in community activities.

Learning from International Models:

While the US system can be strengthened in these areas, it's beneficial to look at models in other countries. The UK, for example, offers a more universal healthcare system through the National Health Service (NHS), providing comprehensive care for seniors, though wait times for certain services can be a challenge. Many European countries offer robust social care programs, including home care assistance, meals on wheels, and community centers, supporting seniors' independence and reducing the burden on family caregivers. These services are often subsidized or publicly funded, making them more accessible to a wider range of individuals. Exploring and adapting successful elements from these international models can inform policy development in the US, leading to a more comprehensive and equitable system of elder care. For instance, the concept of "social prescribing" in the UK, where healthcare providers refer individuals to community-based programs and activities to address social isolation and improve well-being, could be a valuable addition to the US system.

By implementing these comprehensive solutions, encompassing legal frameworks, planning initiatives, and addressing social determinants of health, we can create a more supportive and compassionate society for our aging population. This requires a collaborative effort involving

Chapter 6: A Call to Action

individuals, families, communities, governments, and organizations working together to protect our elders and promote their well-being, ensuring they live with dignity and receive the care and support they deserve.

The Elderly Crisis

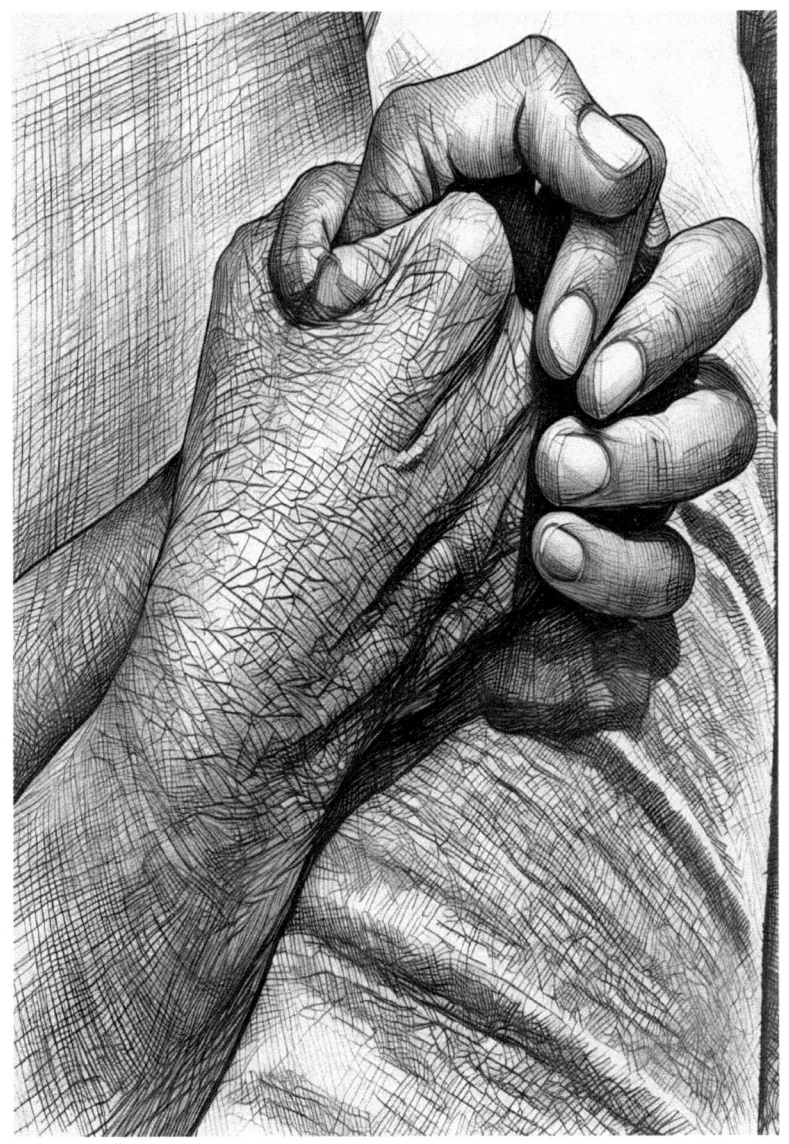

Chapter 7

Coming Together: Creating a Supportive World for Seniors

Creating a truly supportive society for our aging population requires a multifaceted approach, with active participation from governments, communities, families, and individuals. It's a shared responsibility that demands commitment and collaboration at every level.

Government's Role: Setting the Foundation for Dignified Aging

Governments play a crucial role in establishing policies and allocating resources that ensure the well-being of seniors. This includes:

Fund Adequate Social Programs: Robust social safety nets are essential for ensuring seniors' basic needs are met.

- **Increase Funding for Medicare, Medicaid, and Social Security:** These programs provide vital support for healthcare, long-term care, and retirement income. However, current funding levels often fall short, leaving many seniors struggling to afford essential services. Increased funding is crucial to expand eligibility, enhance benefits, and address the growing demand for elder care services. For example, expanding Medicare coverage to include dental, vision, and hearing care can significantly improve seniors' quality of life.

- **Invest In Affordable Housing Options:** The rising cost of housing poses a significant challenge for many seniors on fixed incomes. Investing in senior-specific housing, including assisted living facilities and senior centers, is crucial. These facilities should offer a range of services, such as meal programs, transportation assistance, and social activities, promoting independence and reducing isolation. Incentivizing developers to build affordable senior housing through tax breaks or zoning regulations can also expand housing options. For instance, co-living arrangements, where seniors share housing and expenses, can be a viable and affordable option.

Implement Supportive Policies: Legislation and regulations can protect seniors' rights and ensure their well-being.

- **Enact and Enforce Legislation Protecting Older Adults from Abuse, Neglect, and Exploitation:** Strong laws with clear definitions of abuse and neglect, coupled with robust enforcement mechanisms, are essential. This includes mandatory reporting requirements for professionals who interact with seniors, such as healthcare providers and financial advisors. Furthermore, providing resources for victims of abuse, such as legal assistance and counseling services, is crucial.

- **Strengthen Anti-Discrimination Laws to Combat Ageism:** Ageism, or discrimination based on age, is a pervasive issue that can limit seniors' opportunities in employment, housing, and social participation. Stronger legal protections against ageism, coupled with public awareness campaigns to challenge negative stereotypes about aging, are needed.

- **Provide Tax Incentives for Employers Who Offer Elder-Friendly Workplace Policies:** Encouraging employers to offer flexible work arrangements, paid family leave, and other benefits that support

Chapter 7: Coming Together

employees who are caring for aging parents can alleviate the burden on caregivers and allow them to balance work and family responsibilities.

Invest in Research and Innovation: Advancements in medical technology and assistive devices can significantly improve seniors' quality of life.

- **Fund Research on Aging-Related Diseases:** Investing in research to understand and treat age-related conditions, such as Alzheimer's disease, Parkinson's disease, and arthritis, is crucial for improving seniors' health and well-being.

- **Develop Innovative Technologies to Assist Older Adults with Daily Living:** Assistive technologies, such as smart home devices, wearable sensors, and robotic companions, can help seniors maintain their independence and safety. Funding research and development in this area can lead to more user-friendly and affordable technologies.

- **Improve Access to Telemedicine Services:** Telemedicine can expand access to healthcare for seniors, particularly those living in rural areas or with mobility limitations. Investing in telehealth infrastructure and training healthcare providers on how to effectively utilize telemedicine technologies is crucial.

How a New Administration Can Make a Difference:

A new administration can prioritize elder care by:

- **Creating a National Strategy on Aging:** Developing a comprehensive plan that addresses the diverse needs of the aging population, including healthcare, housing, long-term care, social services, and economic security.

- **Establishing a Dedicated Agency or Task Force**

on Aging: This entity would be responsible for coordinating federal programs and policies related to aging, as well as conducting research and providing public education on elder care issues.

- **Increasing Funding for Programs that Support Seniors and Caregivers:** This includes programs like Meals on Wheels, the National Family Caregiver Support Program, and the Eldercare Locator.
- **Promoting Age-Friendly Communities:** Providing grants and incentives to communities that implement policies and programs that make their cities and towns more livable for seniors.

Community's Role: Building a Network of Support

Communities play a vital role in creating inclusive and supportive environments for seniors; this includes fostering intergenerational connections through shared activities and programs, developing age-friendly infrastructure such as accessible transportation and walkable neighborhoods, supporting local organizations that provide services and social engagement opportunities for older adults, promoting volunteer programs that engage seniors and connect them with the wider community, establishing community gardens and shared spaces that encourage social interaction and physical activity, raising awareness about the needs and contributions of seniors to combat ageism, and creating opportunities for lifelong learning and skill-sharing among all age groups.

- **Foster Intergenerational Connections:** Bridging the gap between generations can benefit both seniors and younger individuals.
  - **Organize Community Events that Bring Together People of Different Ages:** Intergenerational programs, such as volunteer opportunities, shared meals, and cultural

exchange programs, can foster mutual understanding and respect.

- **Develop Age-Friendly Communities:** Creating communities where seniors can thrive is essential.
  - **Make Communities More Accessible for Older Adults:** Improving infrastructure, such as sidewalks, ramps, and public transportation, can make it easier for seniors to get around and participate in community life.
  - **Create Safe and Inclusive Spaces for Older Adults:** Senior centers, community centers, and parks should be designed to be accessible and welcoming to seniors, providing opportunities for social interaction and recreation.
- **Support Local Organizations:** Grassroots organizations are often at the forefront of providing direct services to seniors.
  - **Support Local Organizations that Provide Services to Older Adults:** Volunteering time or donating resources to organizations that offer services such as meal delivery, transportation assistance, and home care can make a significant difference in the lives of seniors.

Family's Role: Providing Love and Care

Families are the cornerstone of elder care, providing essential support and companionship; this includes offering practical assistance with daily tasks, providing emotional support and reducing isolation, respecting their autonomy and dignity, and actively planning for future care needs.

The role of family in the lives of elders is undeniably paramount, fostering a profound sense of security and safety through protection, assistance, and guidance. For our mother, every aspect of her care was unequivocally family-driven. We, her children, provided comprehensive emotional and physical support; we shared responsibilities such as bathing, Stephen managed grocery shopping, and I handled laundry and daily needs, while we both attended medical appointments together. This unwavering commitment ensured that our mother felt completely secure and prioritized, receiving everything she needed without hesitation. Even now, following her passing, our family remains closely knit, continuing to support one another whenever and wherever a need arises.

- **Open Communication:** Discussing aging and caregiving needs openly and honestly is crucial.
    - **Have Open and Honest Conversations About Aging, Caregiving Needs, and End-of-Life Wishes Within Families:** These conversations can be difficult, but they are essential for ensuring that seniors' wishes are respected and that family members are prepared for the challenges of caregiving.
- **Provide Practical Support:** Assistance with daily tasks can significantly improve seniors' quality of life.
    - **Help with Daily Living Tasks, Errands, Transportation, and Emotional Support:** Providing practical assistance with everyday tasks, such as grocery shopping, laundry, and transportation, can help seniors maintain their independence. Offering emotional support and companionship is equally important.
- **Respect Autonomy and Dignity:** Treating seniors with respect and valuing their autonomy is paramount.
    - **Respect the Autonomy and Independence**

of Older Adults While Providing Appropriate Support: It's crucial to balance the need to provide care with the desire to respect seniors' independence and decision-making abilities.

A Global Perspective:

The challenges of aging populations are not unique to the United States. Many countries around the world are grappling with similar issues. Learning from international best practices can inform policy development and program implementation. For example, countries like Sweden and Denmark have comprehensive social welfare programs that provide extensive support for seniors, including home care, long-term care, and financial assistance. Japan, with its rapidly aging population, has implemented innovative programs to promote active aging and community engagement for seniors. Sharing knowledge and collaborating on solutions can help countries around the world build more supportive and inclusive societies for their aging populations. Ultimately, creating a world where seniors can age with dignity and security requires a global commitment to action.

The Elderly Crisis

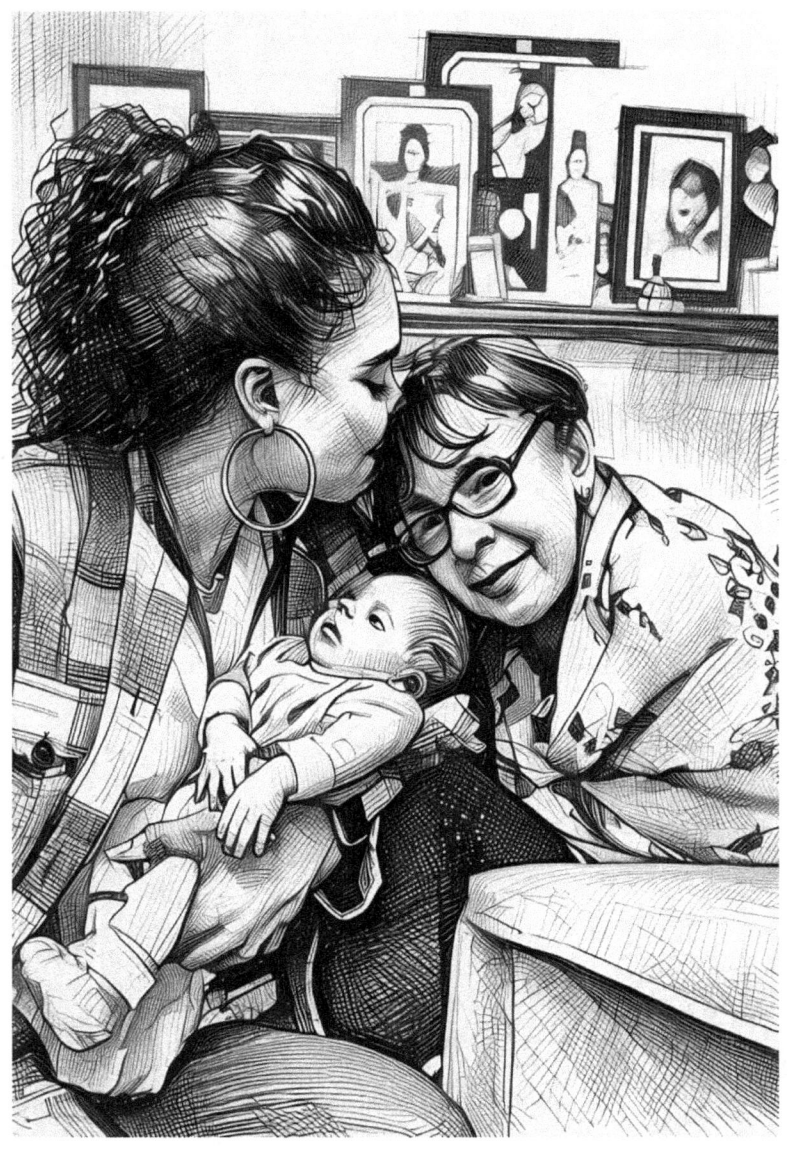

Chapter 8

Our Legacy of Love: Building a World Where No Elder Stands Alone

Leaving a Legacy of Care and Support: Building a Better Future for Generations

Leaving a legacy that positively impacts future generations is a multifaceted endeavor. It requires a conscious effort to address environmental concerns, contribute to social well-being, provide educational and financial support, uphold strong ethical principles, and preserve personal and family history. Each of these elements plays a vital role in shaping a better world for those who come after us.

The Environment's Impact on the Elderly: A Critical Consideration

The environment plays a crucial role in the health and well-being of the elderly. Seniors are particularly vulnerable to environmental hazards due to a variety of factors, including weakened immune systems, pre-existing health conditions, and reduced mobility.

- **Air Pollution:** Poor air quality can exacerbate respiratory illnesses, such as asthma and COPD, which are more prevalent among older adults. Exposure to pollutants can lead to increased hospitalizations and even premature death.

- **Extreme Weather Events:** Heatwaves, floods, and other extreme weather events pose significant risks to seniors. They may have difficulty regulating their body temperature during heatwaves, increasing their risk of heatstroke. Reduced mobility can make it challenging to evacuate during floods or wildfires.

- **Access to Green Spaces:** Exposure to nature has numerous health benefits, including reduced stress, improved mental health, and increased physical activity. Limited access to green spaces can negatively impact seniors' physical and mental well-being.
- **Food Security:** Environmental degradation and climate change can disrupt food production and distribution, leading to food insecurity. Seniors with limited mobility or financial resources may be particularly vulnerable to food shortages.

Therefore, environmental stewardship is not just an abstract concept; it's a critical component of ensuring the health and well-being of our aging population.

1. Environmental Stewardship: Protecting Our Planet for Future Generations

- **Reduce Your Carbon Footprint:** Minimize your environmental impact by adopting sustainable practices in your daily life. This includes reducing energy consumption through energy-efficient appliances and lighting, conserving water by fixing leaks and using water-saving fixtures, and choosing sustainable transportation options like walking, biking, or public transport.

- **Support Environmental Causes:** Donate to environmental organizations working to protect our planet. Advocate for strong environmental protection policies at the local, state, and national levels. Participate in local conservation efforts, such as tree planting or community cleanups.

- **Pass on Environmental Values:** Educate children and grandchildren about environmental issues and inspire them to become environmental stewards.

Encourage them to adopt sustainable practices in their own lives and empower them to become advocates for environmental protection.

2. Social and Community Impact: Building a More Just and Inclusive Society

- **Volunteer Your Time:** Dedicate time to community service, mentoring young people, or assisting those in need. Volunteering not only benefits others but also provides a sense of purpose and fulfillment.

- **Support Local Businesses and Organizations:** Patronize local businesses committed to sustainable practices and ethical labor standards. Support non-profit organizations working to address social issues, such as poverty, homelessness, and inequality.

- **Foster Intergenerational Connections:** Build relationships with younger generations, sharing your wisdom and experiences while learning from their perspectives. Mentoring young people can provide them with guidance and support, helping them to develop into responsible and compassionate adults.

3. Financial and Educational Support: Investing in Future Generations

- **Invest in Education:** Support educational initiatives, such as scholarships, school programs, or libraries. Education is a powerful tool for breaking the cycle of poverty and creating opportunities for future generations.

- **Plan for Charitable Giving:** Consider establishing a charitable trust or making planned gifts to organizations that align with your values. This can create a lasting legacy of support for causes you care about.

- **Pass on Financial Literacy:** Teach children and

grandchildren about financial responsibility, saving, and investing. Equipping them with the knowledge and skills to manage their finances wisely will contribute to their future economic security.

My mother's life stands as a powerful testament to these very principles, a vibrant embodiment of how profoundly one individual can cultivate opportunities and nurture care across generations. Throughout her journey, her belief in these ideals transcended mere sentiment; she actively poured her very essence into the lives of others. Her commitment to education wasn't confined to institutional support; it was about igniting the flame of potential within individuals through the tangible act of funding scholarships, directly contributing towards people's tuitions, and generously supporting church-led educational initiatives – deeply understanding that education serves as the fundamental bedrock upon which future generations can dismantle cycles of poverty and build brighter futures.

Her approach to charitable giving transcended mere transactions; it was a heartfelt investment in the causes that resonated with her deepest values. By thoughtfully pouring into charitable trusts and making planned gifts, she wasn't just donating; she was weaving a tapestry of enduring support, ensuring her compassion would continue to touch lives long after her time. This wasn't just about giving; it was about creating a lasting echo of her empathy in the world.

And in passing on financial literacy, she wasn't just sharing dry facts; she was igniting a spark of economic empowerment within her fellow co-workers, colleagues, friends, children, and grandchildren. By weaving tales of financial responsibility, instilling the discipline of saving as a cornerstone of future freedom, and unlocking the potential of investing, she was laying a solid foundation for our enduring security and independence. This wasn't merely about managing figures; it was about bestowing the very keys to self-sufficiency, illuminating our individual pathways toward a future brimming with stability and prosperity.

Because my mother lived these principles so fully, her legacy extends far beyond her own years. She cultivated a garden of opportunity, nurtured it with generosity, and ensured its fruits would continue to blossom in the lives of her community and the broader society. Her actions demonstrate that a life lived with intention and a heart directed towards the well-being of others can indeed create an enduring and deeply meaningful legacy – a legacy that my brother, Stephen, has embraced with remarkable dedication. He has not only absorbed her financial acumen but has also become a conduit for her continued generosity, ensuring that not a holiday, celebration or birthday passes without those close to our family feeling the warmth of his memory, a tradition he carries forward with the same spirit of giving that defined our mother. He ensures that her charitable endeavors continue to flourish, and he has, with both eloquence and genuine care, taken it upon himself to maintain the personal connections she so valued. Stephen's example has profoundly shaped my own understanding of the power of giving and the importance of extending a helping hand, a trait I deeply admire and one that has become a guiding principle for our family. On this past Mother's Day, as we visited her resting place, we also made it a point to visit our aunt, to offer her the customary flowers and spend time in remembrance and gratitude. It is Stephen who, in many ways, embodies the characteristics and values of our mother, particularly in his approach to financial stewardship, healthcare advocacy, and the unwavering principles by which he lives. His commitment ensures that her legacy of compassion continues to enrich our lives and the lives of those around us.

4. Ethical and Moral Compass: Leading by Example

- **Live with Integrity:** Demonstrate strong ethical principles in all your interactions and decisions. Be honest, fair, and compassionate in your dealings with others.

- **Promote Peace and Justice:** Advocate for social justice and work towards a more equitable and inclusive society. Stand up for the rights of others and challenge injustice wherever you see it.

- **Leave a Positive Impact:** Strive to make a positive difference in the lives of others, whether through acts of kindness, mentorship, or simply by being a positive role model.

5. Documenting Your Legacy: Sharing Your Story with Future Generations

Preserving and documenting family history is essential for connecting future generations to their roots. It provides a sense of identity, belonging, and continuity.

- **Share Your Stories:** Share your life experiences, values, and wisdom with family and friends through stories, letters, or memoirs. Your personal narrative can provide valuable lessons and inspiration for those who come after you.

- **Preserve Family History:** Document family history, traditions, and values for future generations. This can include creating family trees, collecting photographs and documents, and recording oral histories.

- **Create a Family Legacy Project:** Initiate a family project that benefits the community, such as a community garden, a scholarship fund, or a volunteer initiative. This can be a meaningful way to honor your family's values and make a lasting contribution to the world.

My mum gifted us her history not just through dates and names, but through the vibrant tapestry of jokes that still make us smile, the warmth of laughter that echoes in our

Chapter 8: Our Legacy of Love

memories, and the timeless lessons that continue to guide our steps. And because she cherished every moment, nothing was truly lost; we also hold the tangible legacy of paperwork and full documentation, a rich chronicle of her family's journey and the remarkable story of her own life. This treasure trove, woven with anecdotes and anchored in fact, is now a precious inheritance for our future generations, a vibrant connection to our roots and a guiding light for the paths ahead.

Closing Summary

As we conclude this journey through the complexities of the elderly crisis, we find ourselves not at an end, but at a beginning. We've explored the systemic failures, the personal heartbreaks, and the urgent need for change. Yet, within these challenges lies the opportunity to build a legacy of care, a future where no elder faces their final years alone. This chapter has illuminated how our actions today, from advocating for policy changes to fostering intergenerational connections and protecting our environment, directly impact the lives of our elders and those who will follow.

The 'who will be there?' question that echoes throughout this book is not merely a plea for assistance; it's a call for transformation. It's a call to recognize that the well-being of our elders is inextricably linked to the health of our communities, the integrity of our systems, and the sustainability of our planet. By embracing environmental stewardship, by building bridges across generations, and by championing ethical and compassionate care, we are not just addressing a crisis; we are laying the foundation for a society that values and protects its most vulnerable.

This "Elderly in Crisis" is more than a collection of stories and statistics; it's a testament to the enduring human spirit and a roadmap for creating a world where every elder is met with dignity, respect, and unwavering support. Let us carry forward the lessons learned, the empathy awakened, and the commitment to action ignited within these pages. Let us be the ones who are there, not just when they need us the most, but always. Let us build a legacy of love and care that will resonate through generations, ensuring that no elder ever stands alone.

This book is a testament to the extraordinary woman my mother, Cecelia Veronica Carby, was. Her influence extends far beyond those who knew her personally. She possessed a rare combination of sharp intellect and boundless empathy. Her wisdom, accumulated through a life rich in experience, was always offered freely, generously illuminating the path for those seeking guidance. She had a profound impact on countless lives, not only through her kindness and generosity but also through her unwavering commitment to making the world a better place. She instilled in me the importance of compassion, resilience, and the power of human connection. Her spirit, her values, and her indelible mark on my life are woven into the fabric of this book. Through these stories and insights, her legacy will continue to inspire and empower, touching lives now and into the future. This book is a tribute to her enduring spirit, a beacon of her wisdom, and a testament to the profound love between a mother and child. Mum, your love continues to guide me, and your memory will forever be a blessing.

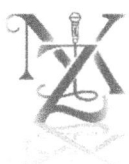